Self-Assessment Colour Review

Respiratory
Medicine

Third edition

Stephen G Spiro

BSc, MD, FRCP
Professor of Respiratory Medicine and
Honorary Consultant Physician, University College Hospital and
Royal Brompton Hospital, London, UK

Richard K Albert

MD
Denver Health Medical Center, Denver, CO, USA

Jeremy S Brown

MBBS, PhD, FRCP
University College London/UCLH Trust
Centre for Respiratory Research, London, UK

Neal Navani

MA, MRCP
University College London/UCLH Trust
Centre for Respiratory Research, London, UK

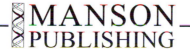
MANSON
PUBLISHING

Copyright © 2011 Manson Publishing Ltd
ISBN: 978-1-84076-139-9

A CIP catalogue record for this book is available from the British Library.

For full details of all Manson Publishing Ltd titles please write to:
Manson Publishing Ltd, 73 Corringham Road, London NW11 7DL, UK.
Tel: +44(0)20 8905 5150
Fax: +44(0)20 8201 9233
Email: manson@mansonpublishing.com
Website: www.mansonpublishing.com

Commissioning editor: Jill Northcott
Project manager: Julie Bennett
Copy editor: Carrie Walker
Design and layout: Cathy Martin
Colour reproduction: Tenon & Polert Colour Scanning Ltd, Hong Kong
Printed by: New Era Printing Company Ltd, Hong Kong

Contents

Preface

One of the pleasures of respiratory medicine is also its greatest challenge – it has so many diseases within its subspecialty area, as well as encompassing many of the problems seen in acute medical practice, that it requires an extensive knowledge of medicine. Judging from the previous editions of this book, learning through the question and answer format has proven popular and attractive. We have completely rewritten this text and included many new cases to discuss. Those which remain have all been reviewed and updated as necessary. All the authors have an extensive international experience of general internal as well as respiratory medicine, and virtually every case is an actual clinical problem or presentation that they have encountered over the last few years.

The book is, in the same way as respiratory medicine, predominantly based on radiological presentations. There is a huge variety of radiological questions, and the reasons for any particular answer are carefully explained. The same applies to the physiological questions, an area absurdly neglected in much of today's teaching and training modules. In order to maintain the reader's interest, there is no particular sequence to the question list, and the reader can dip in and out, select a topic from the index, or just work through the book. All the main topic areas are covered: radiology, physiology, infection, malignancy, interstitial lung disease, diseases of the pleura, immunology and immunosuppression, respiratory complications of systemic diseases, hereditary conditions, sleep-disordered breathing, asthma, chronic obstructive pulmonary disease, respiratory failure, and problems around the intensive care unit. If you answer all the 200 or so questions and understand their meaning, this book, intended for trainees as well as general physicians, will, we hope, have enhanced your knowledge of respiratory medicine. And if you have enjoyed this style of education as much as we have enjoyed putting the book together, we will have succeeded in our task.

Stephen G Spiro
Richard K Albert
Jeremy Brown
Neal Navani

Classification of cases

All references are to question and answer numbers

Thoracic oncology
6, 19, 22, 31, 34, 39, 41, 55, 66, 86, 96,
97, 99, 104, 107, 117, 128, 132, 133,
136, 139, 147, 149, 152, 153, 154, 157,
169, 176, 177, 178, 189, 191, 199

Lung infections
7, 13, 14, 17, 18, 33, 36, 42, 44, 48, 54,
56, 62, 64, 71, 72, 73, 76, 79, 89, 95,
100, 102, 103, 105, 110, 113, 116, 120,
127, 130, 131, 134, 156, 185, 186, 188,
194, 203, 204

Airways disease
1, 2, 5, 11, 28, 45, 47, 78, 106, 112,
121, 126, 129, 137, 144, 145, 150, 167,
173, 174, 193, 200

Interstitial lung disease
4, 8, 15, 25, 30, 40, 53, 57, 67, 80, 92,
94, 109, 124, 125, 135, 140, 142, 143,
151, 165, 168, 170, 180, 184, 190, 197

Pleural disease
3, 20, 24, 26, 29, 37, 45, 46, 58, 70, 74,
82, 83, 202

Sleep medicine
16, 63, 85, 111, 115, 159, 164, 171, 179

Respiratory physiology
23, 27, 43, 59, 68, 69, 77, 91, 93, 98,
101, 108, 114, 119, 141, 146, 148, 158,
160, 161, 181, 192

Pulmonary vascular disease
12, 49, 52, 60, 84, 183

Respiratory complications of systemic
diseases
38, 73, 75, 81, 90, 155, 162, 163, 182

Chest wall disease
21, 51, 87, 122, 146

Miscellaneous
9, 10, 32, 35, 40, 50, 61, 65, 88, 118,
123, 138, 166, 172, 175, 187, 195, 196,
198, 201

Abbreviations

ACE	angiotensin-converting enzyme	HIV	human immunodeficiency virus
ADH	antidiuretic hormone		
AIDS	acquired immune deficiency syndrome	HPOA	hypertrophic pulmonary osteoarthropathy
ANCA	antineutrophil cytoplasmic antibody	HRCT	high-resolution computed tomography
ARDS	acute respiratory distress syndrome	INR	International Normalized Ratio
BAL	bronchoalveolar lavage	K_{CO}	carbon monoxide transfer coefficient
BCG	Bacille Calmette-Guérin		
BiPAP	bi-level positive airway pressure	LAM	lymphangioleiomyomatosis
		LEMS	Lambert–Eaton myasthenic syndrome
BMI	body mass index		
BO	bronchiolitis obliterans	LIP	lymphocytic interstitial pneumonitis
BTS	British Thoracic Society		
CAP	community-acquired pneumonia	MDI	metered dose inhaler
		MRC	Medical Research Council
CFTR	cystic fibrosis transmembrane regulator	MRI	magnetic resonance imaging
		OSA	obstructive sleep apnoea
CMV	cytomegalovirus	$PaCO_2$	arterial partial pressure of carbon dioxide
CNS	central nervous system		
COPD	chronic obstructive pulmonary disease	PaO_2	arterial partial pressure of oxygen
CPAP	continuous positive airway pressure	PAS	periodic acid–Schiff
		PAVM	pulmonary arteriovenous malformation
CRP	C-reactive protein		
CSF	cerebrospinal fluid	PCR	polymerase chain reaction
CT	computed tomography	PEFR	peak expiratory flow rate
DL_{CO}	diffusing capacity of the lung to carbon monoxide	PET	positron emission tomography
DPI	dry powder inhaler	PiO_2	inspired partial pressure of oxygen
EAA	extrinsic allergic alveolitis		
EBUS	endobronchial ultrasound	RQ	respiratory exchange ratio (quotient)
ECG	electrocardiograph		
ELISA	enzyme-linked immunosorbent assay	RV	residual volume
		SaO_2	arterial oxygen saturation
ESR	erythrocyte sedimentation rate	TB	tuberculosis
		TLC	total lung capacity
FEV_1	forced expiratory volume in 1s	VATS	video-assisted thoracoscopic surgery
FiO_2	fraction of inspired oxygen		
FRC	functional residual capacity	VC	vital capacity
FVC	forced vital capacity	VO_2max	maximal oxygen uptake
GINA	Global Initative for Asthma	V/Q	ventilation/perfusion
GOLD	Global Initiative for Chronic Obstructive Lung Disease		

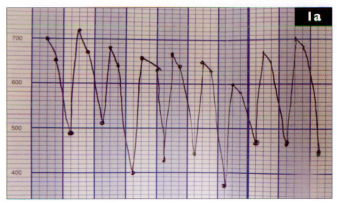

1 i. What is the investigation shown in **1a**?
ii. How should the patient be managed?

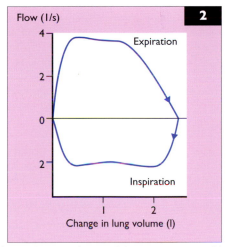

2 This flow–volume loop (**2**) was obtained from a 56-year-old patient with marked respiratory distress and an audible wheeze in whom the initial diagnosis was 'status asthmaticus'. The patient had recently been discharged from hospital after 4 weeks of treatment in intensive care for ARDS.
i. What does the flow–volume loop demonstrate?
ii. What is the likely diagnosis?
iii. What inhalation treatment might be helpful?

| **1b** REDUCE | | | | INCREASE |

←——————————————————————————→

TREATMENT STEPS

Step 1	Step 2	Step 3	Step 4	Step 5
	asthma education			
	environmental control			
as needed rapid-acting ß$_2$-agonist	as needed rapid-acting ß$_2$-agonist			

CONTROLLER OPTIONS

	SELECT ONE	SELECT ONE	ADD ONE OR MORE	ADD ONE OR BOTH
	low-dose ICS*	low-dose ICS *plus* long-acting ß$_2$-agonist	medium- or high-dose ICS *plus* long-acting ß$_2$-agonist	oral glucocorticosteroid (lowest dose)
	leukotriene modifier**	medium- or high-dose ICS	leukotriene modifier	anti-IgE treatment
		low-dose ICS *plus* leukotriene modifier	sustained-release theophylline	
		low-dose ICS *plus* sustained-release theophylline		

* inhaled glucocorticosteroids   ** receptor antagonist or synthesis inhibitors

1 i. This is the daily PEFR measurement. Measurements are lowest in the early morning and highest in the afternoon as all individuals show at least a 10% diurnal rhythm for peak flow. In asthma, this is exaggerated, and a more than 20% diurnal variability is consistent with a diagnosis of asthma.
ii. Patients with asthma should be managed according to a stepwise regime (e.g. GINA; **1b**). They should be started at the most appropriate step for their symptoms and moved up when their asthma is uncontrolled and down when it is well controlled.

2 i. The flow–volume loop demonstrates a reduction in the maximum inspiratory and expiratory flows, which both plateau over a large proportion of the FVC manoeuvre and a low FVC <3 l. The reduction in flow is more marked during inspiration, and this is typical of narrowing of the extrathoracic trachea.
ii. The initial diagnosis of asthma should be avoided on the basis of the physical signs, which, in addition to stridor, are most marked in inspiration but often audible during expiration. A simple test to detect upper airway obstruction is the ratio of FEV_1 to peak flow, i.e. FEV_1 (ml)/PEFR (l/min). This is usually less than 10, but in upper airway obstruction the peak flow is affected most, e.g. 2000 ml ÷ 150 l/min = 13.

The data would also be compatible with a high tracheal or laryngeal area of narrowing/collapse, as after a tracheostomy.

Another cause of this presentation is a high tracheal tumour, which, because of its slow onset, may mimic asthma. However, the wheeze will be fixed and the symptoms constant, unlike in asthma.
iii. A mixture of oxygen (21%) and helium (79%) as helium is less dense than nitrogen, allowing a greater flow of gas.

3 A 74-year-old male has previously worked as a plumber and has been exposed to asbestos. He has not previously had any respiratory problems and now has a chest X-ray (3) before an elective hip replacement.
i. What does it show?
ii. What further action is required?
iii. How else can asbestos exposure affect the lungs?

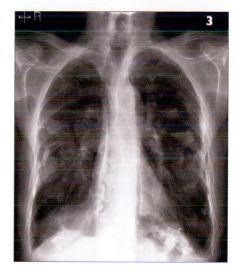

4 This 65-year-old male has a 4-month history of a dry cough and exertional breathlessness.
i. Describe the appearances on HRCT (4).
ii. What clinical features might you expect to find on examination?
iii. What are the associations and complications of this condition?
iv. What is the treatment?

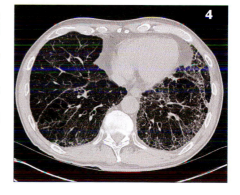

3 i. The chest X-ray demonstrates extensive pleural plaques. These are evident both above the hemidiaphragms and also along the ribs throughout the thorax.

ii. This is a benign condition and rarely causes symptoms. The plaques occur after a latent period of approximately 20–40 years following asbestos exposure and almost exclusively involve the parietal pleura. Plaques may grow over time, but as they are not considered premalignant no further action is required.

iii. Asbestos may affect the lung in several ways (*Box*).

> **Asbestos-related pulmonary manifestations**
> * Pleural plaques
> * Benign pleural effusion
> * Diffuse pleural thickening
> * Rounded atelectasis (Blesovsky sign)
> * Asbestosis (pulmonary fibrosis)
> * Mesothelioma
> * Non-small-cell lung cancer

4 i. The HRCT axial cut demonstrates reticular opacities, traction bronchiectasis, and honeycombing in a subpleural and basal distribution. Honeycombing is recognized by the presence of one or more rows of clustered cysts (<5 mm in diameter) and implies a poor prognosis. The features are characteristic of idiopathic pulmonary fibrosis. HRCT is a very reliable method of making the diagnosis, and lung biopsy (which would demonstrate usual interstitial pneumonitis) is not required in most cases.

ii. The examination features would include digital clubbing (25–50% of cases) and fine end-inspiratory 'Velcro-like' crackles at the bases. The pansystolic murmur of tricuspid regurgitation, a raised jugular venous pressure, and peripheral oedema may herald the development of pulmonary hypertension.

iii. No cause for idiopathic pulmonary fibrosis has been discovered. It may, however, be associated with connective tissue diseases (e.g. rheumatoid arthritis, scleroderma and mixed connective tissue diseases) and in this context has a better prognosis. The condition is linked to an increased incidence of lung cancer and is a cause of respiratory failure and secondary pulmonary hypertension. The 5-year survival is worse than for many extrathoracic cancers, at 20–40%.

iv. The treatment options are limited. A combination of *N*-acetylcysteine, prednisolone, and azathioprine is recommended to reduce the rate of decline of lung function, although it does not improve mortality. Lung transplant is rarely performed for patients with idiopathic pulmonary fibrosis, since most patients present over the age of 60 (the cut-off for transplantation in the UK).

5 i. Describe this chest X-ray (**5**) of a 74-year-old smoker.
ii. How would you judge the severity of the condition?

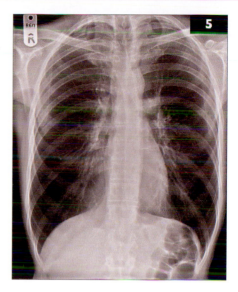

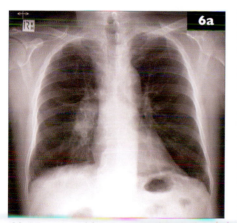

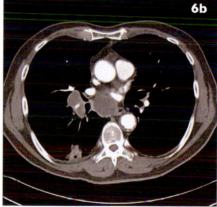

6 i. How would you stage this patient's lung cancer (**6a, 6b**)?
ii. How reliable is CT for identifying metastatic mediastinal disease?
iii. What is the maximum size of so-called normal nodes on CT scanning?

COPD severity	GOLD criteria (2008) FEV$_1$ % predicted	National Institute for Health and Clinical Excellence criteria (2004) FEV$_1$ % predicted
Mild	>80%	50–80%
Moderate	50–80%	30–49%
Severe	30–49%	<30%
Very severe	<30% or <50% with chronic respiratory failure	–

5 i. The posteroanterior chest X-ray shows hyperinflated lung fields, flattening of the diaphragms, a general reduction in lung density, and a peripheral pruning of vascular markings consistent with COPD.
ii. The severity of COPD is most usefully assessed by spirometry. The GOLD (Global Initiative for Chronic Obstructive Lung Disease) guidelines define COPD from when the post-bronchodilator FEV$_1$/FVC ratio is <0.7 (*Table*).

Other factors that predict the prognosis and exacerbation rate include transfer factor for carbon monoxide, breathlessness (according to the MRC scale), exercise capacity, BMI, PaO_2, and cor pulmonale.

6 i. The chest X-ray (**6a**) shows a large right hilar mass and no obvious primary tumour. The primary tumour may be resectable, but only if there is no mediastinal disease present. A CT of the thorax and upper abdomen should be performed (**6b**). Such a CT scan in fact has shown the primary tumour behind the hilar mass, sitting in the apical segment of the right lower lobe. It is cavitating, suggesting a squamous cell lesion. The CT scan confirms the hilar nodal enlargement and also shows enlarged subcarinal nodes, making the patient almost certainly inoperable. In otherwise operable cases of non-small-cell lung cancer, liver metastases are seen on CT in 5% and adrenal deposits in 7% of patients.
ii. CT scanning gives a 30–40% false-positive and also a false-negative rate, and is therefore much less reliable than a PET scan, which has a specificity of 85–90% for identifying tumour.
iii. The maximum size of 'normal' nodes on a CT scan is 10 mm in the node's short axis, although this will be falsely negative in up to 40% of cases, particularly with adenocarcinomas.

7 The photomicrograph (**7**) shows a Gram stain of sputum expectorated by a 19-year-old male with symptoms of fever, rigors, and a productive cough of 2 days' duration. He has experienced four episodes of radiographically documented pneumonia and numerous episodes of acute otitis media and sinusitis in the past.

i. What does the Gram stain show?

ii. What is the most likely diagnosis?

iii. What additional diagnostic considerations are raised by this clinical presentation?

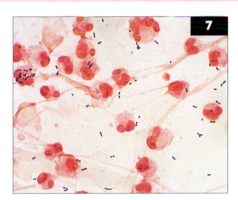

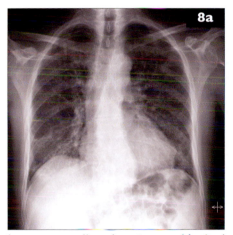

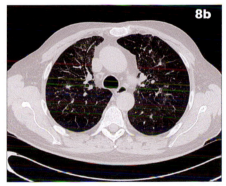

8 This 50-year-old male presented with gradually progressive dyspnoea over the course of 6 months. His mother had become unwell at that time, and he had started visiting her daily to look after her. Her chest X-ray (**8a**) is shown.

i. Describe the appearances seen on the HRCT (**8b**) of the lungs.

ii. What important history would you obtain?

iii. What is the likely diagnosis?

iv. How would you treat this condition?

v. What is the differential diagnosis of bilateral upper lobe shadowing?

7 i. The sputum Gram stain shows numerous polymorphonuclear leukocytes, strands of mucus, and many Gram-positive, lancet-shaped diplococci. Refractile capsules are evident on many of the bacteria.

ii. The young patient has an acute pneumococcal pneumonia and has suffered numerous recurrent respiratory infections.

iii. Most patients with recurrent respiratory infections have no identifiable host defect. However, recurrent pneumonias in the same lobe or segment should suggest an anatomical abnormality. When multiple sites have been involved, disorders of mucociliary clearance such as cystic fibrosis or the ciliary dyskinesia syndrome (Kartagener's syndrome) are an important consideration.

Recurrent infections with encapsulated organisms such as the pneumococcus are consistent with a defect in opsonization (e.g. complement, IgG or IgG subtype deficiencies). Deficiencies of complement components are rare and are best managed by immunization and by the early treatment of infectious complications.

Immunoglobulin deficiencies can also be primary (inherited) or acquired due to acquired B-cell disorders, medications, or intercurrent illnesses. IgA is heavily concentrated in mucosal secretions, where it inhibits bacterial adherence. Although selective IgA deficiency is common, it rarely results in serious respiratory infection unless other deficiencies coexist. IgG deficiency (either generalized or restricted to subclasses IgG1 and IgG3) predisposes to more frequent and more severe respiratory infections. Intravenous immunoglobulin replacement may be helpful.

8 i. The HRCT (**8b**) shows diffuse ground-glass shadowing with some areas of centrilobular nodularity. The chest X-ray (**8a**) shows a mainly upper lobe nodular infiltrate.

ii. Ask about exposure to any pets or unusual dusts or chemicals. In this case, the patient had had a cockatoo that he had been feeding since his mother had become unwell. Budgerigars and pigeons are common causes of this, as are the classical irritants encountered in farmer's lung, bark-stripper's lung, etc.

iii. EAA or hypersensitivity pneumonitis may be caused by exposure to a variety of dusts and antigens, and may be confirmed by avian precipitins in the serum and removal of the source, i.e. the bird. A careful occupational history is essential.

iv. Patients must be instructed to avoid the allergen or precipitant. Oral prednisolone may be used during the initial few weeks until the patient feels better, although there is no definite evidence on optimal dose and duration.

v. The differential diagnosis includes sarcoidosis, pneumoconiosis, ankylosing spondylosis, and TB.

9 i. How does a pulse oximeter work?

ii. The accuracy of most pulse oximeters decreases below what percentage saturation?

iii. What factors affect the accuracy of pulse oximetry?

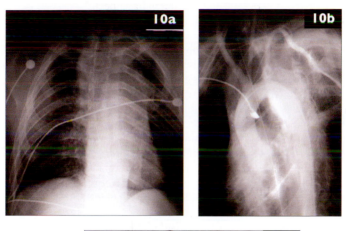

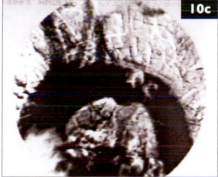

10 A 24-year-old male motorcyclist was admitted as an emergency having been involved in a road traffic accident.

i. What abnormality can be seen on the plain chest radiograph (**10a**), and what diagnosis must be suspected?

ii. What is demonstrated on the subsequent vascular imaging films (**10b, 10c**)?

iii. Where is this lesion normally encountered, what is the mechanism of injury, and what are the possible consequences?

9 i. A pulse oximeter is a spectrophotometer that measures the absorption of light at two wavelengths, one in the infrared range at a wavelength of 940 nm (absorbed by oxyhaemoglobin) and the other at a wavelength of 660 nm (absorbed by reduced haemoglobin).The absorption at these two wavelengths is compared, and the percentages of oxygenated and reduced haemoglobin are calculated. The pulse oximeter compares absorption measured during systole and diastole and uses the difference to reflect only the absorption of arterial blood, thereby limiting errors induced by absorbance in venous blood and other tissues.

ii. The accuracy of most oximeters decreases below 75% saturation. Above this level, the accuracy is approximately 4%.

iii. Standard pulse oximeters are unable to distinguish dyshaemoglobins, most notably carboxyhaemoglobin and methaemoglobin, from oxyhaemoglobin. In smoke inhalation, pulse oximetry reflects absorption by both oxyhaemoglobin and carboxyhaemoglobin, and thus may overestimate the true oxygenation status. Any factor that affects assessment of the arterial pulse (e.g. motion, low-perfusion states) may distort the reading. Specific light sources, such as fluorescent or infrared lamps, can cause erroneous signals if the oximeter probe is not shielded. Dark skin pigmentation and darker coloured nail polishes can also interfere with light transmission, thereby lowering oximeter readings.

10 i. There is gross widening of the mediastinum on the plain chest radiograph (**10a**), even allowing for the anteroposterior nature of the examination. The severity of the injury and the mediastinal widening make traumatic aortic transection a definite possibility.

ii. The aortogram (**10b**) shows a bulge in the region of the distal aortic arch/proximal descending aorta. This is clearly shown on digital subtraction angiography (**10c**) to be due to disruption of the aortic wall.

iii. This lesion is characteristically seen at the aortic isthmus, i.e. the junction between the aortic arch and the descending aorta. This injury is believed to occur because the arch can move forward with deceleration whereas the descending aorta is relatively fixed. Immediate exsanguination will occur in many cases. Those individuals who reach hospital can undergo repair of the ruptured segment, usually with the insertion of a short length of prosthetic graft. Spinal cord ischaemia can occur either before or during surgery, with consequent lower limb paralysis.

11 i. What has been done to this patient whose chest X-ray (**11**) is shown here, and why?

ii. How would the patient have presented?

iii. What are the potential risks of the treatment?

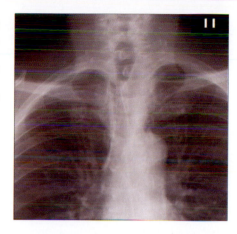

12 This 72-year-old female presented with a 3-month history of malaise, sweats, weight loss, cough, and occasional haemoptysis. She developed a pneumonia that was treated with antibiotics but responded poorly, and she remained unwell with a low-grade fever. She was mildly anaemic with an ESR of 120 mm in 1 hr and a CRP value of 92 mg/l.

i. What does the radiograph (**12**) show, and what is the differential diagnosis?

ii. How would you make the correct diagnosis?

iii. How would you treat the patient?

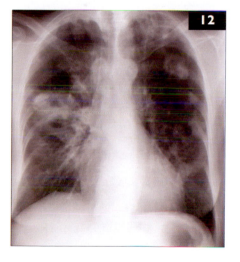

11 i. The image shows an endotracheal stent. Stents are deployed for the management of extrinsic compression of an airway.

ii. The most likely cause of tracheal compression is a retrosternal goitre, and the patient would have presented with stridor. However, this should be managed surgically and not with a stent. Malignant masses or lymph nodes are the most common cause of more distal main airway compression and may need stenting. Although airway stents are an effective initial treatment, definitive management of the underlying lesion should be first choice, for example using surgery (although this is unlikely as the disease is usually advanced by the time major airway occlusion occurs). Radiotherapy and chemotherapy can be effective, especially in small-cell lung cancers. However, in tracheal cancers and squamous cell lung cancers, where the disease often relapses locally after chemotherapy and radiotherapy, stents can dramatically relieve symptoms.

iii. Airway stents also may become a nidus of infection and may become blocked due to secretions, resulting in a sudden deterioration in respiratory status.

12 i. The chest radiograph shows multiple lesions of variable size throughout both lung fields, most of which have cavitated. The differential diagnosis includes staphylococcal pneumonia, lymphoma, TB, cavitating squamous cell carcinoma, and a vasculitis – most likely Wegener's granulomatosis.

ii. This female had Wegener's granulomatosis. The diagnosis was made by identifying cytoplasmic ANCA in high titre in the peripheral blood. This is positive in more than 90% of cases and negative in classic polyarteritis nodosa and other vasculitides. The titres of cytoplasmic ANCA parallel disease activity and return to normal when the disease is in remission. They can predict reactivation if a rise is detected in patients in remission.

iii. Untreated disease is fatal, with a median survival of 5 months. The treatment of Wegener's granulomatosis, whether confined to the lung or more extensive with renal involvement, is with prednisolone and cyclophosphamide. In general, prednisolone is given at 1 mg/kg for 4 weeks and then slowly tailed down to a maintenance of 10 mg/day. Cyclophosphamide is commenced at 100–150 mg orally, and is then reduced by 25 mg every 2–3 months to 50 mg/day. Treatment is continued for 1 year after remission has been achieved.

Approximately 75% of patients achieve a complete remission, and a further 15% a partial remission. Serial cytoplasmic ANCA titres should be performed to predict relapse, which can occur in up to 50% of cases. The prognosis is better for Wegener's granulomatosis that is confined to the lung.

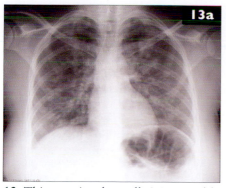

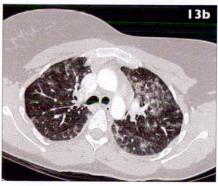

13 This previously well 36-year-old East African female has had increasing shortness of breath for 3 weeks associated with a dry cough and some retrosternal chest pain on deep breathing. On examination, she is pyrexial at 37.7°C and cyanosed, with a respiratory rate of 40 breaths/min. Auscultation of the chest reveals some fine bilateral crepitations, and blood and sputum cultures are both negative. Her chest X-ray (**13a**) and CT scan (**13b**) are shown.
i. What is the likely diagnosis?
ii. How can the diagnosis be confirmed, and what is a likely underlying condition?
iii. What is the recommended treatment?

14 Shown here (**14**) is a swollen right ankle and diffuse macular rash in a young female with cystic fibrosis.
i. What is the diagnosis?
ii. What is the medical treatment and prognosis?

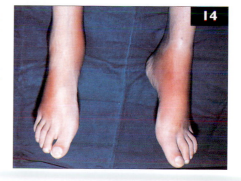

13 i. The combination of an insidious but progressive illness with cough, marked hypoxaemia, and a chest radiograph showing bilateral perihilar infiltrates with peripheral sparing (**13a**) (confirmed as mainly upper lobe symmetrical ground-glass infiltrates with peripheral sparing on CT scan (**13b**)) are highly suggestive of *Pneumocystis jirovecii* pneumonia (formerly *Pneumocystis carinii* pneumonia or PCP). In addition, the patient belongs to a high-risk population (sub-Saharan African).

ii. *P. jirovecii* pneumonia is the classical opportunistic pneumonia affecting HIV-positive patients, especially once their lymphocyte CD4-positive count has fallen to less than 200 cells/µl. Presentation is usually a slow onset of dyspnoea associated with an unproductive cough, sometimes associated with a distinctive retrosternal pain on inspiration or coughing. The pyrexia is relatively mild, and chest signs are often limited. Patients characteristically have a fall in oxygen saturations on exercise and a marked reduction in their carbon monoxide transfer factor.

Diagnosis requires obtaining a BAL or induced sputum sample for cytology, in which the characteristic cysts can be identified by cytology using Grocott's methenamine silver staining (which stains the cysts black), or immunofluorescence with specific antibodies. A classical presentation in someone known to be HIV positive can be treated empirically, reserving invasive investigations for if the patient fails to respond. *Pneumocystis jirovecii* pneumonia also occurs in patients with other T-cell defects such as those who have had organ or bone marrow transplantation, or individuals on long-term immuosuppression.

iii. Treatment is with high-dose co-trimoxazole (120 mg/kg in divided doses daily for 3 days, and then 90 mg/kg). If the PaO_2 is <9.3 kPa (70 mmHg) or the alveolar oxygen gradient is >4.7 kPa (33 mmHg), adjuvant corticosteroids have been shown to improve outcome (e.g. 40 mg prednisolone twice a day for 5 days, followed by 40 mg for 5 days and then 20 mg for 11 days). For patients who are intolerant of Septrin (co-trimoxazole), second-line therapy is usually primaquine 15 mg once daily and clindamycin 600 mg four times a day.

14 i. The illustration shows a diffuse vasculitis involving the skin and synovium. Vasculitis of the skin may also be nodular or purpuric (without thrombocytopenia). It is associated with severe pulmonary disease and chronic *Pseudomonas aeruginosa* infection. It has been attributed to an overspill into the systemic circulation of immune complexes resulting from the hyperimmune stimulation associated with chronic pulmonary disease.

ii. Medical treatment consists of short-term, high-dose oral steroids. This will usually produce complete resolution. Immunosuppressive agents have been used, but experience with them is limited.

15 A 40-year-old male presented with a 3-week history of cough, malaise, and fevers that had not responded to a variety of broad-spectrum antibiotics. His blood tests showed an ESR of 115 mm/hr, a CRP of 194 mg/l and a white cell count of $15.3 \times 10^9/l$ (22% eosinophils at $3.5 \times 10^9/l$). Microbiological tests, including sputum and blood cultures, serology for parasitic infections, and analysis of sputum and faeces for parasites, were all negative. His chest X-ray is shown here (**15a**).

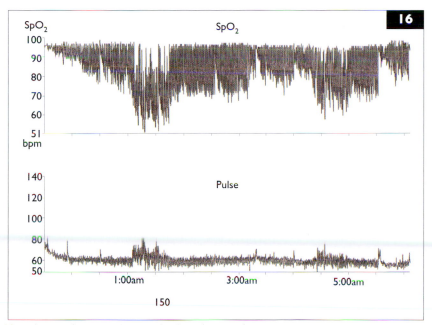

i. The chest X-ray has a characteristic appearance suggestive of which disease?
ii. How can the diagnosis be confirmed?
iii. What is the treatment and prognosis?

16 i. What is this test (**16**), and what does it show?
ii. How useful is this type of study in sleep-disordered breathing?

15 i. The chest X-ray shows patchy
dense consolidation affecting the lung
peripheries, with sparing of the medial
aspects of the lung. These appearances
were confirmed by the CT scan of the
thorax (**15b**). This is highly suggestive
of an eosinophilic pneumonia, an
idiopathic disorder characterized by
eosinophilic infiltration of the lung
parenchyma. Acute (develops over days)

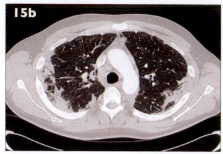

and chronic (develops over weeks or months) forms occur, but the characteristic
peripheral shadowing is most associated with the chronic form.
ii. The blood eosinophil count is not always raised, especially early in the disease,
but BAL fluid will contain a high proportion of eosinophils (usually >25%, but
90% is not uncommon with pulmonary eosinophilia), and this confirms the
diagnosis. Blood IgE levels are usually elevated. Other lung diseases associated with
blood eosinophilia are Löffler's syndrome (transient pulmonary infiltrates often
associated with parasitic infections such as *Ascaris* or *Strongyloides*), or drugs such
as aspirin [aminosalicylic acid] and sulphonamides [sulfonamides]), allergic
bronchopulmonary aspergillosis, Churg–Strauss syndrome, and idiopathic
hypereosinophilic syndrome. Asthma is also frequently associated with a mild
eosinophilia.
iii. Eosinophilic pneumonias usually respond rapidly to oral corticosteroids, with
a complete resolution of symptoms and radiological abnormalities within 1 month
on tapering courses of oral prednisolone starting at between 30 and 60 mg/day.

16 i. The test is an overnight recording of SaO_2 and heart rate.
ii. The equipment will calculate the number of oxygen dips of >4% and give an
hourly dip rate, which will identify sleep apnoea. This is an effective and simple
screen test for OSA and can easily be carried out by the patient at home. It does not
record snoring or actual sleep. It is useful for central apnoea and also for assessing
the requirement for domiciliary oxygen in hypoxaemic patients, such as those with
severe COPD. If the results are not clear cut, a more sophisticated sleep study is
required.

17 This is the chest X-ray (**17**) of a 16-year-old male who presented with a 3-week history of a dry cough and fevers.
i. What does the chest X-ray show?
ii. What is the likely diagnosis?
iii. What contact tracing procedures should be instigated?

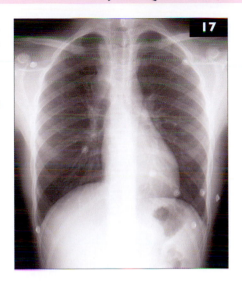

18 This 65-year-old female has rheumatoid arthritis, and her physician wishes to commence immuno-suppression. There is, however, a concern over reactivating a latent TB infection. A tuberculin skin test is positive, and a gamma-interferon test is negative.
i. Describe the chest X-ray (**18**).
ii. How would you interpret the other results?
iii. Does the patient require antituberculous therapy?

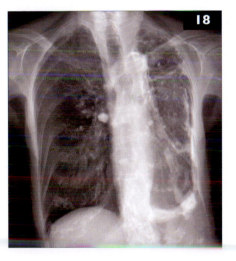

17 i. Unilateral enlarged paratracheal lymph nodes.

ii. Primary pulmonary TB. The initial infection with *Mycobacterium tuberculosis* in children with no prior history of exposure to the disease leads to a small primary focus of infection, usually in the middle to lower zones on the chest X-ray when visible, and associated with enlarged mediastinal nodes on the affected side. The mycobacteria disseminate into the blood from the enlarged nodes and can therefore be seeded throughout the body, but they have a predilection for areas of relatively high oxygen tension such as the apices of the lungs, the CNS, and the metaphyses of the long bones.

Primary disease causes symptoms in only a minority of patients (less than 10%), usually resolves spontaneously (often leaving a tuberculoma), and is associated with conversion to a positive tuberculin skin test after 6 weeks. However, primary disease can be complicated by progressive local disease within the lungs, bronchial obstruction by enlarged nodes (especially the middle lobe, leading to bronchiectasis), bronchogenic TB due to the rupture of a caseating node into the bronchial tree, pleural or pericardial effusions, miliary TB, and tuberculous meningitis.

iii. Contact tracing is initiated to identify (a) cases who have caught TB from the index case, (b) the potential source of infection for the index case, and (c) other patients who may have been infected by this source. Recommendations vary between countries but usually suggest the screening of all subjects who live with the index case and other close contacts such as school classmates.

Screening requires a clinical history, chest X-ray, and tuberculin skin testing (at least in children or those who have not been given the BCG vaccine). The new gamma-interferon blood tests for TB identify whether the patient has circulating lymphocytes that recognize an antigen specific for *M. tuberculosis*, and may provide a more specific and sensitive test for identifying infected patients than tuberculin skin testing.

18 i. The chest X-ray shows calcified lymph nodes and volume loss on the left, with marked, very thick calcified pleura indicating previous TB infection.

ii. The positive tuberculin skin test is in keeping with previous TB infection but may also occur following BCG vaccination and in patients with latent or active TB. The gamma-interferon test is specific for TB infection and is not usually positive in patients who have had a BCG. The test is raised in patients with latent TB infection.

iii. Taking the above answers into account, this patient has evidence of previous TB infection but no latent TB, and she will not require TB prophylaxis prior to immunosuppression.

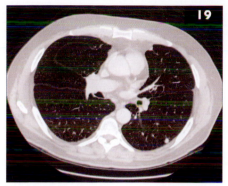

19 i. Describe the CT image (**19**) of this 65-year-old male who is a heavy smoker.
ii. How should this be managed?

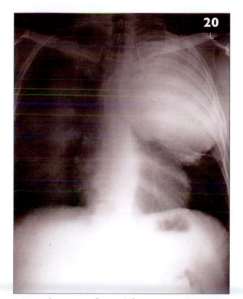

20 A 57-year-old non-smoking male, with no respiratory symptoms, began to behave in an uncharacteristically aggressive and uninhibited manner early in the morning. What is the likely cause of the radiographic shadow (**20**), and what is the explanation for his behaviour?

Nodule size (mm)*	Low-risk patient[†]	High-risk patient[‡]
≤4	No follow-up needed[§]	Follow-up CT at 12 mo; if unchanged, no further follow-up[‖]
>4–6	Follow-up CT at 12 mo; if unchanged, no further follow-up[‖]	Initial follow-up CT at 6–12 mo then at 18–24 mo if no change[‖]
>6–8	Initial follow-up CT at 6–12 mo then at 18–24 mo if no change	Initial follow-up CT at 3–6 mo then at 9–12 and 24 mo if no change
>8	Follow-up CT at around 3, 9, and 24 mo, dynamic contrast-enhanced CT, PET, and/or biopsy	Same as for low-risk patient

* Average of length and width. [†] Minimal or absent history of smoking and of other known risk factors. [‡] History of smoking or of other known risk factors. [§] The risk of malignancy in this category (<1%) is substantially less than that in a baseline CT scan of an asymptomatic smoker. [‖] Non-solid (ground-glass) or partly solid nodules may require longer follow-up to exclude indolent adenocarcinoma.

19 i. The CT scan demonstrates a 7 mm nodule in the left lower lobe with background changes of emphysema.
ii. The causes of this nodule include malignancy (primary or secondary) or benign causes such as past or current infection. In order to distinguish malignant from benign nodules, the Fleischner Society have published guidelines (*Table*) on the management of solitary pulmonary nodules, taking into account the relatively slow doubling time of lung cancer.

20 Massive pleural fibroma, with spontaneous hypoglycaemia. The huge size of the tumour in an otherwise healthy patient suggests that it is benign in nature. The diagnosis is easily confirmed by percutaneous needle biopsy. Large mesenchymal tumours may produce insulin-like growth factors. It is probable that these peptides both stimulate the growth of the tumour itself, which may attain great size, and lead to spontaneous hypoglycaemia. Insulin-like growth factors are normally produced under the control of growth hormone, and their abnormal production leads to its suppression by a negative feedback mechanism. Plasma insulin and C-peptide levels are also low. Despite their large size, the tumours can be removed quite easily surgically as they usually arise from the parietal pleura on a finger-like stalk. Resection leads to complete resolution of the biochemical abnormalities.

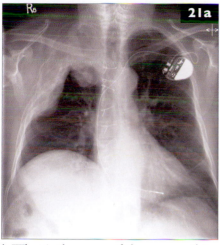

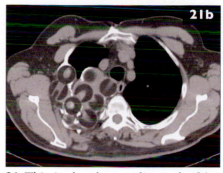

21 This is the chest radiograph (**21a**) and CT scan (**21b**) of the thorax of a 78-year-old male who has presented with a minor haemoptysis. He was treated for TB in the 1950s.

i. What is the cause of the most striking finding?
ii. What was this a treatment for, and what other operative therapies are there for this disease?

22 This male presents having had right anterior chest pain for 1 month.
i. What is the abnormality on the chest X-ray (**22**)?
ii. Which cell type of lung cancer is most commonly associated with this complication, and what test is best for recognizing this?
iii. How would you treat the symptoms?

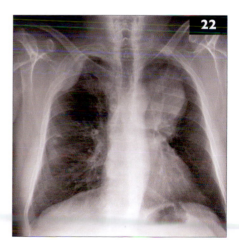

21 i. The CT scan shows that the patient has previously been treated with plombage – the insertion of inert balls made of Leucite extrapleurally inside the chest. These collapse the underlying lung.

ii. Plombage was a surgical therapy for TB used before antibiotic therapy was available. Other surgical treatments included crushing of the phrenic nerve (which leaves a small supraclavicular scar and a raised hemidiaphragm on the treated side) and thoracoplasty, in which the ribs over the upper lobe were removed. All these treatments collapsed the underlying lung and controlled TB by making the affected lobe underventilated and therefore hypoxic (as *Mycobacterium tuberculosis* requires aerobic conditions to grow). Antituberculous chemotherapy now means these operations are generally obsolete, although thoracoplasty may very rarely be used to control highly drug-resistant TB.

Nowadays, the main relevance of these surgical treatments are the long-term complications. Thoracoplasty causes a restrictive lung function impairment which can lead to type 2 respiratory failure that responds well to chronic nocturnal non-invasive ventilation, and plombage can become infected or cause pressure effects on local structures.

22 i. The chest X-ray shows a mass destroying the right third rib and an associated soft tissue mass. There is a large tumour mass in the left upper lobe. The patient had presented with chest pain, and a non-small-cell lung cancer was diagnosed at bronchoscopy. Small-cell lung cancers most commonly develop bony metastases in up to 40% of patients, but they can occur in any cell type. The bony lesion is usually lytic, i.e. destructive, but tissue masses of tumour can grow out from the bony lesion, as in this case. The vertebral bodies are another common site for this.

ii. Bone lesions are usually identified at staging, although the great majority present with symptoms of pain, bone tenderness, and an elevated serum alkaline phosphatase, or serum calcium if extensive. The PET scan has surpassed isotope bone scanning and CT scanning as the most useful test to identify these lesions.

iii. If the lesion is solitary and painful, a single fraction of radiotherapy is effective in 70–80% of cases. This can be repeated as necessary. Analgesia should follow the pain ladder, starting with paracetamol and a non-steroidal anti-inflammatory medication. This can be increased to opiates, initially short acting to assess dose requirement, and then to slow-release preparations with short-acting top-ups as necessary. It is important to administer antinausea medication as necessary and to add aperients to prevent predictable constipation.

23 Patient A has a large left pleural effusion and a single breath gas transfer factor (DL_{CO}) of 55% of normal, along with a transfer coefficient (K_{CO}) that is 90% of normal. Patient B with bullous emphysema has a DL_{CO} of 55%.
i. What is the K_{CO}? How is it measured?
ii. Why does the K_{CO} in Patient A correct to near normal?
iii. What is the K_{CO} likely to be in Patient B (i.e. high, normal, or low), and why?

24 This is the chest radiograph (**24**) of a 30-year-old male who is aysmptomatic apart from mild dyspnoea on exertion.
i. What does the chest radiograph show?
ii. What are the possible causes?
iii. What should the lung function tests show?
iv. What is the management?

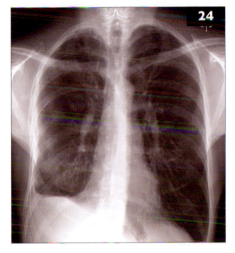

Lung function results

FEV_1	2.7 (65% expected)
FVC	3.8 (61% expected)

23 i. The K_{CO} is the single breath gas transfer factor (DL_{CO}) corrected by the alveolar volume. The alveolar volume is measured by an inert gas technique – usually using helium – which is inspired together with the carbon monoxide. As the helium is inert, it will not escape from the lungs, and the dilutional decrease measured on expiration will give the alveolar volume, that is, the volume of lung that saw the helium and therefore the carbon monoxide. In other word, it is the amount of volume that was available in the circumstances of this test for gas exchange. The DL_{CO} divided by the alveolar volume gives the transfer coefficient, which is the quality of gas exchange in those areas of the lungs that were available to the two gases.

ii. The K_{CO} in Patient A corrects to near normal as the alveolar volume is essentially that of the non-affected lung, i.e. the right lung, which will exchange gas normally.

iii. Here, the K_{CO} is likely to be low. In a patient with emphysema, the DL_{CO} will be low because of poor ventilation and perfusion balance due to parenchymal damage. The lung volumes, however, will be normal or larger than normal, and the alveolar volume will be normal or high. Correcting a low DL_{CO} by a normal or high alveolar volume will give a low K_{CO}. This low (often very low) K_{CO} is characteristic of emphysema.

24 i. The chest radiograph shows marked pleural thickening affecting the right hemithorax.

ii. The likely causes of unilateral pleural thickening are previous empyema, TB, or haemothorax on the affected side. In addition, pleural tumours, in particular mesothelioma, can cause pleural thickening, which would be progressive and usually associated with pain and pleural effusions. Benign asbestos-related pleural disease is usually bilateral. Rarer causes include radiotherapy or drug reactions (e.g. practolol, methysergide, dantrolene, methotrexate, and drugs associated with a lupus-like syndrome such as procainamide, isoniazid, and hydralazine).

iii. The lung function tests should show a restrictive defect with reduced lung volumes and a normal transfer factor. In this patient, the FEV_1 was 2.7 (65% of predicted) and the FVC 3.1 (61% of predicted), giving a ratio of 87%.

iv. Benign pleural thickening requires no further investigation, and there is no specific treatment except for surgical removal of the pleura. However, surgery is difficult due to the dense adhesions of pleura to the lung, and it is reserved for when the physiological effects of the pleural thickening are severe. Over several months, initially quite marked pleural thickening after empyema or haemothorax can often undergo a significant degree of resolution without intervention. Progressive pleural thickening needs to be biopsied (either CT-guided or VATS) to exclude the presence of tumour.

25 A 72-year-old female presented with a several week history of increasing shortness of breath and dry cough. She had recently been admitted for management of cardiac failure and atrial fibrillation but was not now in cardiac failure. On examination, she was apyrexial and had fine inspiratory crepitations in both lung fields. Blood and sputum cultures were negative, and blood tests including white cell count were unremarkable except for a CRP of 34 mg/l.

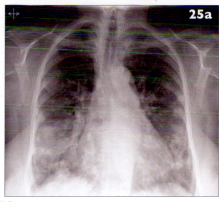

i. Describe the radiological appearances (25a).
ii. What is the differential diagnosis, and what specific questions in the history are important?
iii. How can the most likely diagnosis for this radiological appearance be confirmed?

26 Shown here is the chest X-ray (26) of a patient who presented with neck swelling that started after a severe coughing fit.
i. What does this chest X-ray show?
ii. What is the likely underlying cause?
iii. How should the patient be managed?

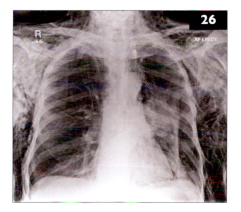

25 i. The chest X-ray (**25a**) shows bilateral peripheral airspace shadowing suggestive of consolidation. The CT scan (**25b**) shows patchy dense peripheral consolidation.

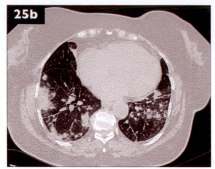

ii. Pneumonia should always be considered as a cause of consolidation, but the long history, lack of systemic symptoms, and normal temperature count against an infective cause in this case. The CT scan appearances are characteristic of an organizing pneumonia, a complication of amiodarone treatment. It can also occur in response to infection, radiotherapy, and chemotherapy, or with no obvious cause (cryptogenic organizing pneumonia). The history should specifically ask about treatment with amiodarone as well as any treatment for cancer. About 5% of patients on amiodarone develop respiratory complications, the incidence being higher in patients receiving more than 400 mg/day. Amiodarone can cause an interstitial pneumonitis, organizing pneumonia (as in this case), or rarely non-cardiogenic pulmonary oedema. Other causes of non-infective consolidation include alveolar cell carcinoma, lymphoma, pulmonary eosinophilia, and vasculitis.

iii. The radiological appearance combined with a history of amiodarone use is usually adequate to make the diagnosis. CT scans may demonstrate that the patches of consolidation and the liver are of relatively high density due to the accumulation of iodine. Lung function tests will show a restrictive defect with a low transfer factor. BAL may recover 'foamy' macrophages containing phospholipids due to the inhibition of phospholipase by amiodarone. Although transbronchial biopsy will only occasionally obtain diagnostic material, a VATS biopsy of organizing pneumonia will show the characteristic budding of fibroproliferative material into the airways. The treatment is to stop amiodarone and start oral corticosteroids (30–60 mg/day, weaning off over several months), which are usually very effective for organizing pneumonia.

26 i. The X-ray shows marked subcutaneous emphysema that is delineating the tissue planes of the soft tissues of the neck and thorax.

ii. A small pneumothorax or pneumomediastinum due to the rupture of alveoli as a consequence of the coughing fit. This is more likely to happen in patients with asthma or COPD.

iii. A CT scan of the thorax may be necessary to identify the pneumothorax or pneumomediastinum. Most cases settle spontaneously without the need for an intercostal drain to control the pneumothorax, or surgical intervention.

27 This 66-year-old male has breathlessness on minimal exertion and is hypoxic at rest. Examination of his chest reveals dry inspiratory crackles. Explain the lung function test abnormalities: FEV_1 50% normal; FVC 55% normal, FEV_1/FVC ratio 95%; TLC 60% normal; FRC 60% normal; RV 80% normal; DL_{CO} 40% normal; K_{CO} 80% normal.

	Pre-bronchodilator	Post-bronchodilator
FEV_1 (l)	2.1	2.5
FEV_1 % predicted	50	60
FVC (l)	3.3	3.5
FEV_1/ FVC %	64	71

28 This spirometry (*Table*) is from a 25-year-old male who complains of a cough at night.
i. What is the diagnosis?
ii. What constitutes a significant bronchodilator response?
iii. What other investigations might be useful?

29 A 75-year-old male presents with this chest X-ray (**29**).
i. What are the most likely causes, and how would you make the diagnosis?
ii. If cytology is negative, what next?
iii. If this proves malignant, what treatment would you suggest?

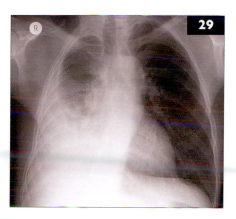

27 The spirometry shows a restrictive defect together with uniformly and greatly reduced lung volumes. This is very suggestive of intrapulmonary disease. In addition, the DL_{CO} is drastically reduced, at 40% of normal. When it is corrected for the lung volume that 'saw' the carbon monoxide for measuring diffusion, the gas transfer partially corrects to 80% of normal. This still, however, means there is intrapulmonary disease, but the lung units that took in the carbon monoxide and helium were 80% efficient. If the low DL_{CO} were due to extrathoracic disease, it would not have been so low, and it would have corrected to normal as the reduced lung volume exposed to the measurement gases would have been exchanging normally in the lung that took in the carbon monoxide/helium mixture.

28 i. The diagnosis is asthma.
ii. A bronchodilator response is significant if the FEV_1 rises by 15% and 200 ml.
iii. Other investigations that are useful in the diagnosis of asthma include peak flow monitoring morning and evening for a period of 2–3 weeks, sputum or blood eosinophil count, intradermal skin prick testing, bronchial challenges (in a specialized laboratory), exhaled nitric oxide, and bronchoscopy (to exclude airway obstruction and for bronchial biopsies that may show Charcot–Leyden crystals). In a young person, a 6-min exercise test of free-range running can induce a post-exercise drop in PEFR of >20%, which is diagnostic.

29 i. A large effusion in an elderly male is likely to be malignant, from either an adenocarcinoma or a mesothelioma. In a female, breast cancer can cause this appearance. The other important cause is TB. Rarer causes include chylothorax, post-traumatic haemothorax, and post-pneumonia empyema, but the patient would then be ill.
ii. The initial step would be aspiration for cytology and bacteriology. In malignancy, cytology is positive in 50–60% of cases. Repeating the procedure hardly improves the yield. If negative, a CT scan may show a pleural tumour, and a guided core biopsy can be carried out.
iii. Treatment of a large malignant effusion should be by a pleurodesis, ideally by VATS and talc pleurodesis. If a diagnosis has not been made prior to VATS, any suspicious area can be biopsied under direct vision. If malignancy is probable, talc can then be instilled.

30 A 30-year-old HIV-positive female presented with a 3-month history of dry cough and dyspnoea on exercise. She had no systemic symptoms. On examination, she looked well and was apyrexial. The only abnormal signs were fine crepitations in the lung bases. Her blood tests were normal, with a CD4-positive cell count within the normal range. Sputum and/or BAL cultures were consistently negative for myco-bacteria, bacteria, respiratory viruses, and *Pneumocystis*. The BAL differential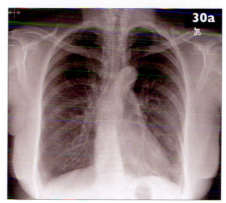
cell count showed 65% lymphocytes. These are the presentation chest radiograph findings (**30a**).
i. Describe the abnormalities of the chest radiograph.
ii. Name six non-infective respiratory complications of HIV infection.
iii. Which are the most likely for this patient?

31 A 60-year-old Caucasian male has a 2-month history of fevers, night sweats, and weight loss.
i. Describe what can be seen in the photograph (**31**).
ii. What is the differential diagnosis?

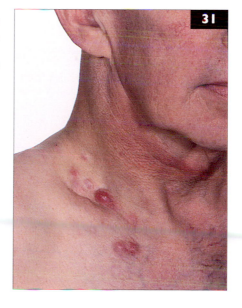

30 i. The chest radiograph shows an asymmetrical nodular consolidation mainly affecting the left lower lobe. CT demonstrated ground-glass shadowing, some small nodules, and thickened interlobular septae.

ii.
- Malignant: Kaposi's sarcoma, lung cancer, pulmonary lymphoma.
- Inflammatory: non-specific interstitial pneumonitis, LIP, organizing pneumonia.
- Other: COPD, bronchiectasis, pulmonary hypertension.

iii. The nodular lung shadowing, and high proportion of lymphocytes in the BAL fluid suggest that the patient has LIP. LIP is characterized by a lymphocytic infiltration of the alveoli and septa, and causes cough and dyspnoea with systemic symptoms in some patients. The diagnosis requires a lung biopsy to exclude other diseases associated with lymphocytic BAL fluid, mainly pulmonary lymphoma, which can have a similar presentation. Treatment is with prednisolone and sometimes chlorambucil, and can be effective. Long-term complications of LIP include lung fibrosis and bronchiectasis.

31 i. The picture shows enlarged cervical lymphadenopathy in the anterior triangle (anterior to the sternomastoid).

ii. The *Table* lists the differential diagnoses.

Differential diagnosis of anterior cervical lymphadenopathy

Infectious
- TB
- Viral, e.g. HIV, Epstein–Barr virus, CMV
- Toxoplasmosis
- Cat scratch disease (*Bartonella henselae*)
- Histoplasmosis, coccidioidomycosis
- Non-tuberculous mycobacteria

Malignancy
- Lymphoma
- Secondaries, e.g. lung, stomach

Reactive
- Secondary to mouth, throat, and local skin infections

Drug reactions, e.g. phenytoin

Sarcoidosis

Langerhans cell histiocytosis

Storage diseases, e.g. Gaucher's disease

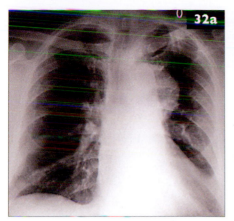

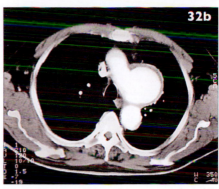

32 A 72-year-old male presented to his GP with a history of hoarseness. Other than moderate hypertension, he had no other past history of note. A radiograph (32a) and CT (32b) were done.

i. What abnormality is present, and what is the likely aetiology?

ii. What classification system can be applied to this abnormality?

iii. Why is the patient hoarse?

iv. How would this condition be managed, and what risks should be discussed with the patient?

33 This is the chest X-ray (33) of a 64-year-old male who has a long history of recurrent chest infections, chronic ear infections, and sinusitis.

i. What does the X ray show, and what is the likely diagnosis?

ii. How is it inherited, and what is the major defect?

ii. How can the diagnosis be confirmed?

iv. What other complications should be discussed with the patient?

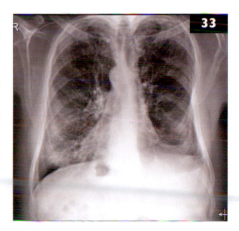

32 i. This patient has a large aneurysm of the aortic arch. The most likely aetiology is hypertension, but serological testing for syphilis would be appropriate. If it had been located at the junction of the arch and descending aorta, a post-traumatic origin would have been a possibility.

ii. Aortic aneurysms may be classified in several ways. A 'true' aneurysm is contained within all the layers of the aortic wall, although these may be greatly thinned and it is common for the aneurysm to be lined with old and new thrombus. Depending on the appearance of the aneurysm, it may be described as 'saccular', as in this case, or 'fusiform' if the dilatation is more cylindrical. If the aneurysm is formed from a localized hole in the aortic wall connecting with a cavity lined only by thrombus, it is described as a 'false' aneurysm. An aortic dissection is often labelled as a 'dissecting aneurysm'. This condition is characterized by the entry of blood into the layers of the aortic wall through a split in the intima with prograde and/or retrograde extension of this process along a variable length of the aorta.

iii. The left recurrent laryngeal nerve has been stretched by the aneurysm.

iv. Hypertension should be controlled and the aneurysm size monitored. If it is static, a conservative approach may be appropriate in someone of moderate general health or advanced age in view of the operative risk. Expansion would dictate surgical excision, probably with replacement of the aortic arch under hypothermic circulatory arrest. The patient should be warned of the magnitude of operative risk (>10% mortality) and specifically advised of the additional risk of perioperative cerebral damage.

33 i. Dextrocardia with some basal bronchial wall thickening. The diagnosis is Kartagener's syndrome – primary ciliary dyskinesia causing recurrent respiratory tract infections, sinusitis, and bronchiectasis, as well as dextrocardia.

ii. Primary ciliary dyskinesia is an autosomal recessive disorder with incomplete penetrance, and occurs in 1 in 15,000–30,000 people in developed countries. Structural defects in ciliary proteins, including the dynein arms, cause the cilia to be immotile. This results in a failure of mucociliary function, mucous collection, and recurrent infections in the lungs and sinuses, with secondary bronchiectasis.

iii. The diagnosis is made by the saccharin test: a small tablet of saccharin is placed in the anterior nares, and the time before the patient experiences a sweet taste is recorded – longer than 40 min suggests ciliary dysfunction. The defect can be confirmed by specialized tests of ciliary movement in nasal mucosal biopsies and/or by electron microscopy of cilial structure. Bronchiectasis can be shown by HRCT.

iv. Many patients suffer from mucous retention in the ear, and most male patients are also infertile and need to be warned about this.

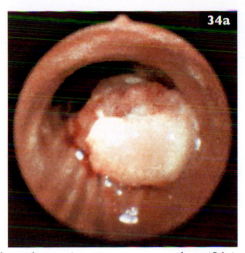

34 i. Describe the bronchoscopic appearances seen here (34a).
ii. What sign would you expect the patient to demonstrate?
iii. Describe the findings of a flow–volume loop from a patient with this condition, and indicate which other conditions may cause a similar flow–volume loop.

35 The mediastinum is divided into three compartments for the classification of mass lesions. The anterior compartment lies between the sternum and the anterior surface of the pericardium and the great vessels. The middle compartment contains the intrathoracic organs and extends to the vertebral column. The posterior compartment comprises the paravertebral spaces. List the more common mass lesions found in each compartment.

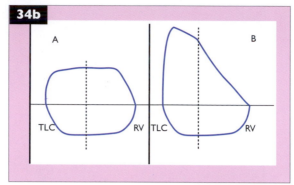

34 i. The image shows a tumour causing obstruction of the trachea. The trachea can be recognized by the presence of cartilaginous rings anteriorly.

ii. The patient is likely to have inspiratory stridor, which can occur with any cause of extrathoracic airway obstruction. Typical flow–volume loops are shown in **34b**. Fixed lesions are characterized by a lack of changes in calibre during inhalation or exhalation, and produce a constant degree of airflow limitation during the entire respiratory cycle. A fixed lesion may be extrathoracic or intrathoracic, and results in a flattening of both the inspiratory and the expiratory portions of the flow–volume loop (**A**). Its causes include post-intubation strictures, goitres, and tracheal tumours.

iii. Variable lesions are characterized by changes in airway lesion calibre during breathing. A variable extrathoracic obstructing lesion results in the limitation of inspiratory flow, seen as a flattening in the inspiratory limb of the flow–volume loop (**B**). During expiration, the air is forced out of the lungs through a narrowed (but potentially expandable) extrathoracic airway. Therefore, the maximal expiratory flow–volume curve may be normal. Causes of variable extrathoracic lesions include glottic strictures, tumours, and vocal cord paralysis.

35

• Anterior: thymoma, thymic carcinoma, thymic cyst, lymphoma, benign or malignant teratoma, seminoma, parathyroid adenoma, retrosternal thyroid goitre, lipoma, leiomyoma, cystic hygroma.

• Middle: lymphoma, benign mediastinal lymphadenopathy, granulomatous diseases (TB, sarcoid), metastatic lymphadenopathy, foregut cysts, oesophageal disorders (achalasia, diverticulae, tumours), aneurysms.

• Posterior: peripheral nerve tumours (schwannoma, neurofibroma, ganglioneuroma), paraspinal abscess, thoracic duct cysts, extramedullary haematopoiesis.

36 A 55-year-old female alcoholic was admitted with high fevers, a cough productive of foul-smelling sputum, and a chest X-ray (**36**).
i. What is the pathological process shown in the chest X-ray?
ii. What organisms are associated with this process, and what are the most likely possibilities in this patient?
iii. What specific investigations are necessary?

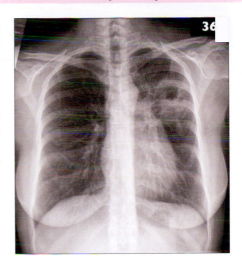

37 A 58-year-old male, with a 4-week history of dysphagia, presented with a short history of vomiting followed by dyspnoea and chest pain. The chest radiograph (**37**) was taken before any intervention. What does it show, and what is the likely cause?

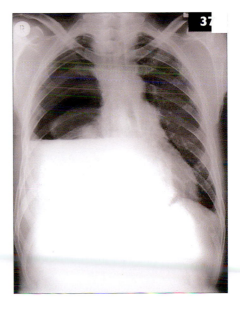

36 i. Cavitation within the left upper lobe, with an air–fluid level present in an area of dense consolidation. The history of fevers and foul-smelling sputum suggests that this is a cavitating pneumonia.

ii. Community-acquired cavitating pneumonias are associated with:
- Anaerobes (associated with aspiration).
- Gram-negative coliforms, including *Klebsiella pneumoniae* (which classically causes an expanding pneumonia in the upper lobe, especially in patients such as alcoholics who have a degree of immunosuppression).
- *Staphylococcus aureus* (usually multiple small cavitations, often occurring after influenza infection).
- 5% of pneumonias due to *Streptococcus pneumoniae*.

On the right patient background or in the right geographical area, other pathogens that cause cavitating lung infections include *Mycobacterium tuberculosis*, non-tuberculous mycobacteria, actinomycosis, *Nocardia*, *Aspergillus*, and other moulds, *Burkholderia pseudomallei* (melioidosis), endemic fungi (e.g. histoplasmosis, coccidioidomycosis), and flukes (paragonimiasis). In addition, septic emboli from infected indwelling lines or right-sided endocarditis will cause multiple cavitating lesions that are often peripheral and associated with effusions.

iii. Microscopy of sputum (including staining for acid-fast bacilli) and cultures of the blood and sputum. Consider a CT scan of the thorax and bronchoscopy to define the cavities in greater detail and to exclude a proximal bronchial lesion causing obstruction to the bronchus supplying the affected lobe.

37 Hydropneumothorax. The presence of a large quantity of both air and fluid in the pleural cavity in a patient with these symptoms is strongly suggestive of rupture of the oesophagus. The fluid was turbid but not purulent. The underlying cause was ulceration of the oesophagus by tuberculous mediastinal lymph nodes.

Rupture of the oesophagus can occur in previously fit individuals, for example after violent vomiting or impaction of a food bolus or foreign body, and is a medical emergency. It may initially cause retrosternal or pleural pain. It may be missed at oesophagoscopy if the tear is small, and is best diagnosed by a barium swallow. Immediate repair by a thoracic surgeon is the treatment of choice.

Rupture can occur as the result of an oesophageal tumour causing necrosis of the wall. This may also occur with a tracheal tumour or metastatic subcarinal nodes. Ensleevement of the lesion with an oesophageal tube can give good palliation.

Other possible causes of hydropneumothorax include the rupture of a large lung abscess, empyema, and the rupture of a tuberculous cavity into the pleural space. Simple aspiration would be inadequate, and drainage with a large-bore intercostal tube is mandatory, together with appropriate intravenous antibiotic therapy.

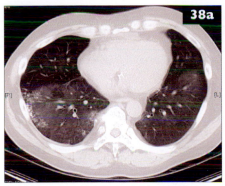 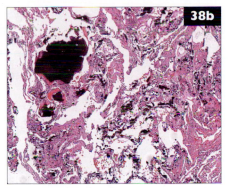

38 A 54-year-old dialysis-dependent male reports progressive dyspnoea on exertion and a dry cough that had their onset 2 years previously, following a 'pneumonia syndrome'. Shown here are his chest CT (38a) and lung biopsy (38b).
i. What does the histology show?
ii. What is the diagnosis?
iii. Which patients are most likely to develop this condition?

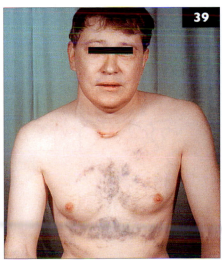

39 i. What is this syndrome (39), and how may it present?
ii. How would you make the diagnosis?
iii. How would you treat this?
iv. Enumerate the presentations of mediastinal involvement by lung cancer.

38 i. The histology shows dense calcium deposits in the lung parenchyma.
ii. Metastatic calcification. In addition to the pulmonary manifestations, it can also affect the heart, stomach, kidney, and lung.
iii. Up to 60–80% of patients on chronic haemodialysis have evidence of metastatic pulmonary calcification on autopsy, most commonly those with secondary hyperparathyroidism and patients with an elevated calcium phosphate product. Less commonly associated diagnoses include primary hyperparathyroidism, multiple myeloma, Paget's disease, hypervitaminosis D, and malignancies.

39 i. This is superior vena caval obstruction, and in an adult (as depicted), lung cancer, small-cell type in particular, is the most likely cause. It is seen in up to 10% of new cases of small-cell tumour. In a younger patient, a lymphoma will be the probable diagnosis. It can present with headaches, especially on bending forward. There will be oedema of the upper limbs and face, especially periorbitally. The oedema can cause a gruff voice and throat pain. The patient may notice the collateral venous pathways in the chest and upper abdomen.
ii. Ultrasound of the neck may identify supraclavicular or scalene nodal enlargement that can be aspirated for cytology under ultrasound. CT scanning will usually show extensive mediastinal nodal masses that are easily accessed by CT-guided biopsy. Failing this, bronchoscopy and biopsy, or EBUS-guided transbronchial biopsy is usually possible and safe.
iii. If the condition is due to small-cell carcinoma, chemotherapy is as effective as radiotherapy, which is the treatment of choice in non-small-cell lung cancer, followed by chemotherapy if the patient is fit enough. Excellent symptomatic relief can be rapidly achieved by a superior vena cava stent provided vascular studies show the superior vena cava to be just compressed and not completely occluded by tumour.
iv. Other presentations of mediastinal involvement include:
- Recurrent laryngeal nerve entrapment in the subaortic fossa.
- Dysphagia due to subcarinal lymph nodes pushing posteriorly into the mid-oesophagus.
- Breathlessness and a high hemidiaphragm due to phrenic nerve entrapment.
- Breathlessness due to atrial fibrillation and/or pericardial involvement, and effusion from invasion by a left lower lobe tumour.
- Horner's syndrome owing to sympathetic chain involvement in the upper mediastinum.
- Chylothorax due to rupture of the lymphatic duct by tumour (more common with lymphoma).

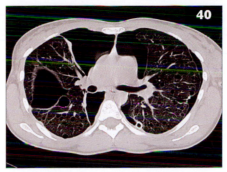

40 A 23-year-old, non-smoking female presented with bilateral spontaneous pneumothoraces. There was no history of illicit drug use. **40** is the CT scan of her thorax.
i. What does the CT scan show?
ii. What is the differential diagnosis of the lung parenchymal appearances?
iii. What other clinical features should be looked for, and what other investigations might be necessary?

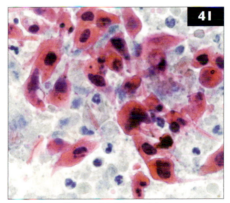

41 This sample (**41**) came from bronchial brushings.
i. What is the abnormality?
ii. What factors determine the sensitivity of bronchial brushing?

40 i. The CT scan shows bilateral tethered pneumothoraces (a drain is also visible posteriorly on the left side). In addition, the lung parenchyma contains multiple thin-walled cysts of varying sizes.

ii. In a young female with a history of pneumothoraces, the CT finding of thin-walled cysts is highly suggestive of lymphangioleimoymatosis (LAM). LAM is restricted to females mainly of child-bearing age, and is characterized by atypical smooth muscle proliferation in the lung (and occasionally mediastinum, retroperitoneal lymphatics, or uterus) causing lung cysts, recurrent pneumothoraces, or chylous effusions. Progression is variable, but respiratory failure occurs in some patients.

In the differential diagnosis, histiocytosis X should be considered but is very unusual in non-smokers and the cysts are usually much more variable in size and shape than in LAM. Bullae and emphysema need to be considered, but the cysts of LAM are too small and central to be bullae and they also have a well-circumscribed wall, unlike emphysematous change. Other diseases associated with cysts include LIP and EAA, but the cysts in these conditions are associated with other parenchyal abnormalities.

iii. LAM can be isolated or associated with about 1% of cases of the autosomally dominant inherited disorder tuberous sclerosis. The clinical features of tuberous sclerosis (subungual fibromas, facial angiolipomas, retinal astrocytomas, renal angiomyolipomas) need to be looked for, and renal imaging may be necessary to identify the renal tumours. The patient's lung function should be measured and usually shows an obstructive defect with impaired gas transfer and gas trapping. The diagnosis is confirmed by lung biopsy, which can be obtained at the same time as surgical treatment of the pneumothoraces is undertaken. Treatment is difficult but mainly involves hormonal manipulation, e.g. intramuscular medroxy-progesterone injections.

41 i. This cytology sample shows large, irregularly shaped cells with prominent nucleoli and coarsely clumped chromatin, indicative of non-small-cell carcinoma. Intercellular bridges, seen as fine parallel lines between cells, correspond to desmosomes and are characteristic of squamous cell carcinoma. The histological feature of keratin pearl formation is not usually visible on cytology specimens. Despite this, experienced cytologists can reliably distinguish squamous cell carcinoma from other types of non-small-cell lung cancer on cytology alone.

ii. The sensitivity of bronchial brushings is primarily determined by whether the lesion that is brushed is visible to the bronchoscopist. Larger, more proximal lesions have a higher yield on bronchial brushing.

42 A previously well 30-year-old female presented to hospital with a 2-week history of dry cough and fevers that had not responded to a 5-day course of amoxicillin. On examination, her temperature was 38°C, she had a respiratory rate of 20 breaths/min, and fine crepitations were audible throughout both lung fields. Her oxygen saturation was 92% breathing air. **42** is her chest radiograph on admission. Her HIV test was negative.

i. What does the chest radiograph show?
ii. What are the most likely organisms for this presentation?
iii. How would you manage this patient?

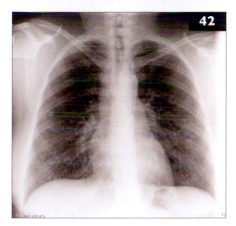

43 A colleague asks for assistance in interpreting the lung volumes measured in the patient whose radiograph is shown here (**43**). The TLC measured by helium dilution was 83% of that predicted, and the RV was 95% of that predicted.

i. How can you explain the normal TLC and RV?
ii. What test would you recommend?

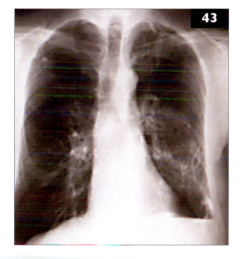

47

42 i. The chest radiograph shows a fine reticulonodular shadowing throughout both lung fields.

ii. The combination of a relatively insidious presentation of an infective respiratory infection with diffuse shadowing would suggest a CAP caused by one of the 'atypical' organisms, especially as there has been no response to amoxicillin. These include *Mycoplasma pneumoniae* and *Chlamydophila pneumoniae*, which together cause around 25% of all cases of CAP (and a higher proportion of the milder cases treated outside hospital), and the rarer organisms *Legionella pneumophila*, *Chlamydophila psittaci*, and *Coxiella burnetii* (the cause of Q fever), which are often grouped with these organisms. Rather than 'atypical', a better term for these bacteria is perhaps 'fastidious' as they are difficult to culture. Although *Mycoplasma* and *Chlamydophila* classically present in this manner, they often also cause a lobar pneumonia that is indistinguishable from *Streptococcus pneumoniae* CAP. *Legionella pneumophila* is one of the three organisms that are the common causes of severe CAP, the other organisms being *Strep. pneumoniae* and *Staphylococcus aureus*.

iii. The patient should have blood and sputum cultures, and should be given oxygen and antibiotics. The important therapeutic point is that atypical/fastidious organisms do not respond to beta-lactam antibiotics but are sensitive to macrolides. As a consequence, most guidelines suggest a combination of beta-lactams and a macrolide as first-line therapy for patients with CAP admitted to hospital. Identification of an atypical infection requires paired serology samples 2 weeks apart, although a single high level of IgM to *Mycoplasma* is enough to confirm *M. pneumoniae* infection. In addition *Legionella* antigen can be detected in the urine if *L. pneumophila* serotype 1 is the cause (70% of *Legionella* cases).

43 i. The TLC and RV appear falsely low because the radiograph suggests larger than normal lung volumes with flat diaphragms. This is a common problem when the helium dilution technique or any other inert gas technique is used to measure lung volumes in the presence of severe airflow obstruction or bullous lung disease. This is because the test does not allow sufficient rebreathing or washout time for the inert gas to enter the poorly ventilated areas of the lung. There is thus often a gross underestimation of the true lung volume. Gas dilution techniques are, however, quite accurate when used in normal subjects or patients without airflow obstruction.

ii. Repeating the measurement of lung volumes using a body plethysmograph will provide much more accurate estimates in patients with airway problems and emphysema. The method has the advantage that it measures the total volume of gas in the lung, including any that is trapped behind closed airways not communicating easily with the mouth. Plethysmography is, therefore, the technique of choice in patients with airflow obstruction.

Results of CSF analysis	
Appearance	Fibrinous
Predominant cell	Lymphocytes
Cell count/mm^3	550
CSF glucose (serum value)	2.1 mmol/l (7.5 mmol/l)
CSF protein	3.1 g/l
Organisms	No organisms seen

44 A 65-year-old has experienced fevers and a change of personality over the last 3 weeks. The results of the CSF analysis are shown in the *Table.*
i. What is the likely diagnosis?
ii. How could the diagnosis be confirmed?

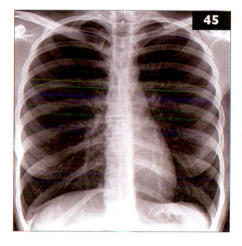

46 i. What is the probable diagnosis of this scan (**46**)?
ii. What is the cause?
iii. What is the possible treatment?

45 A 23-year-old male has a history of asthma and has presented to the Accident & Emergency department following a sudden onset of severe breathlessness.
i. What does the chest X-ray (**45**) show?
ii. What should be the management?

44 i. The results show a lymphocytic meningitis with a low CSF glucose and a very high protein level. This is consistent with tuberculous meningitis.

ii. Organisms are rarely seen on specific staining of CSF for acid-fast bacilli. Culture for *Mycobacterium tuberculosis* is also often negative, and the diagnostic yield may be improved by requesting PCR for *M. tuberculosis*. Other causes of a lymphocytic CSF include listeriosis, cryptococcosis, and sarcoid. HIV testing is recommended for all patients with TB.

45 i. The chest X-ray shows a right-sided pneumothorax, a complication of asthma.

ii. Treatment should be with high-flow oxygen and an intercostal chest drain. High-flow oxygen as well as an intercostal tube is recommended as pure oxygen may help to flush away the inert nitrogen, which constitutes 80% of room air, from the pleural space.

46 i. Malignant mesothelioma. The scan shows generalized pleural thickening of an irregular nature around the left lung and involves the mediastinum. The tumour will also grow into the lung fissures. The differential diagnosis includes adenocarcinoma, but these usually cause irregular growth and pleural masses without the uniformity of mesothelioma.

ii. Around 70% of patients will have a history of exposure to asbestos. Typical occupation groups include plumbers, shipyard workers, boilermen, and sometimes demolition workers. Partners can occasionally be exposed from workers returning home in affected clothing. Crocidolite, which is an amphibole (straight) fibre and can easily penetrate through the tissues, is responsible for 90% of cases. About 1,800 cases a year are seen in the UK, with an expected peak incidence in 2020.

iii. Treatment remains controversial. Surgical resection is a very occasional option in early disease but requires an extensive operation in terms of an extrapleural pneumonectomy. There is little evidence that this is superior to other treatments or to simply best supportive care, with a median survival of 19 months. Radiotherapy is useful for treating diagnostic aspiration or VATS sites to prevent tumour growing through the chest wall. Although chemotherapy is widely used, it may produce a partial response in only 20% of cases. A recent trial of pemetrexed (Alimta) with cisplatin recorded a doubling of response rate compared with cisplatin alone (41% versus 17%) and better median survival times (12.1 versus 9.3 months). Chemotherapy should only be considered in good performance status patients.

47 A 20-year-old patient is complaining of severe breathlessness after each time he roller-blades. The result of exercise testing revealed is shown in **47**.

i. What does the exercise test show?

ii. What is the diagnosis?

iii. How would you manage this condition?

iv. What is the pathogenesis of this condition?

v. What drugs are allowed by the Olympic committee before competition?

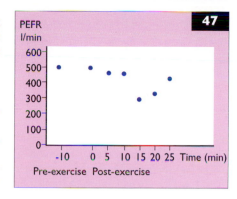

48 This chest radiograph (**48**) is of a 51-year-old male from south-east Asia with dyspnoea and leg swelling. He was jaundiced and had jugular venous distension and ascites on physical examination.

i. What are the radiographic findings?

ii. What infection could account for both the clinical and the radiographic abnormalities?

iii. How can this diagnosis be established?

iv. How is it treated?

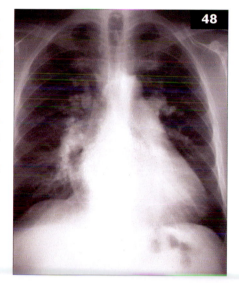

47 i. A 40% fall in peak flow reading after exercise compared with the pre-exercise value.

ii. Exercise-induced asthma. This diagnosis requires a minimum change of 25% in PEFR from the pre-exercise value to the lowest measurement – usually found 10–20 min post-exercise. During exercise, a rise in PEFR is commonly seen.

iii. Advise the patient to inhale a beta-agonist 15 min before exercise and to warm up adequately.

iv. Exercise results in isocapnic hyperventilation and an inhalation of cold air, which results in water loss from the airway lining, causing airway cooling and hypertonicity. These result in vasoconstriction, mast-cell activation, and stimulation of the neural reflexes that cause rebound vasodilatation, oedema, and bronchial hyperreactivity. Mucosal thickening and smooth muscle contraction will then occur, leading to bronchoconstriction of the airways. Current research shows that leukotrienes may also play an important role in exercise-induced asthma.

v. Beta-agonists and sodium cromoglicate (cromolyn).

48 i. The chest radiograph shows enlargement of the pulmonary arteries, suggesting pulmonary hypertension.

ii. The combination of pulmonary hypertension and hepatic failure should suggest the diagnosis of schistosomiasis when the patient originates from an area in which this infection occurs. Schistosomiaisis is caused by one of the blood flukes *Schistosoma mansoni*, *S. japonica* or *S. haematobia*, which are endemic to tropical areas with an appropriate intermediate host population of freshwater snails.

Free-swimming cercariae penetrate human skin and then become schistosomulae that migrate through the lungs to mature in specific mesenteric venous plexuses. Pulmonary manifestations including cough and wheezing, and infiltrates can accompany the systemic symptoms of 'Katayama fever' during the migration of schistosomulae through the lungs in acute schistosomiasis.

Eggs produced by the mature flukes are carried downstream from the mesentery and lodge in the liver. A massive and inappropriate granulomatous inflammatory response to the schistosomal eggs then results in tissue injury and fibrosis. The liver eventually becomes cirrhotic, and portosystemic collateral channels permit embolic eggs to reach the lungs, where a similar inflammatory response ensues. The end result is pulmonary hypertension and cor pulmonale.

iii. The diagnosis of schistosomiasis is based on identification of the eggs in the stools or urine of patients with a compatible clinical presentation and a history of travel or residence in an endemic area (parts of South America, the Caribbean, Africa, and the Middle and Far East).

iv. Treatment with praziquantel is effective in preventing further egg production but may not improve the lesions.

Test	Result	Reference range
FiO_2	0.5	–
pH	7.54	7.35–7.45
$PaCO_2$	3.7 kPa	4.6–6.0 kPa
	(28 mmHg)	(35–46 mmHg)
PaO_2	9.1 kPa	12–16 kPa
	(69 mmHg)	(91–122 mmHg)
HCO_3	18 mmol/l	22–30 mmol/l

49 These arterial blood gas tensions (*Table*) are from a 25-year-old male with nocturnal confusion 24 hr after the pinning of a fractured femur sustained in a motor vehicle accident. No abnormality was detected on physical examination or chest radiography. What is the likely diagnosis and management?

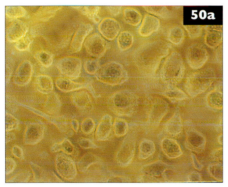
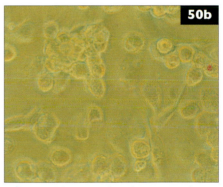

50 Shown here (**50a**) is a photomicrograph of normal human alveolar macrophages obtained by BAL and incubated *in vitro*. **50b** shows the same cell preparation after it has been incubated with gamma-interferon.
i. What are the primary functions of alveolar macrophages?
ii. What are the roles of the secretory products of alveolar macrophages?

49 Fat embolism syndrome. Acute lung injury arises due to a deposition of fat globules displaced from the marrow of the fractured bone into the pulmonary arteries, with a subsequent release of free fatty acids. The syndrome begins with tachypnoea very soon after the trauma or orthopaedic surgery. Chest radiographs may initially be normal but may progress to show a pattern of ARDS, at which time chest examination will reveal widespread fine crackles.

Treatment is with oxygen and is supportive, as for any other form of acute lung injury. Corticosteroids are of no benefit, except possibly if given early. Other features of the syndrome include CNS effects ranging from mild disorientation to seizures and coma, usually 12–36 hr after injury. Petechiae may be present, particularly in the conjunctivae and over the upper extremities and axillae. Both of these features are the result of microvascular injury.

50 i. Alveolar macrophages are the resident phagocytic cells in the lung. They serve as scavengers of inhaled particulate material and senescent cells, and are the sentinels against invasion of the lung by infectious agents.

ii. Non-specific scavenger receptors permit the alveolar macrophage to bind and ingest inert substances without initiating an inflammatory response. In contrast, the ingestion of infectious pathogens typically stimulates a brisk response that results in macrophage activation and inflammatory cell recruitment. These events are regulated by networks of secretory products, primarily cytokines. Gamma-interferon, produced by lymphocytes, is a potent macrophage-activating factor. The alveolar macrophage can also be activated by autocrine cytokines, including tumour necrosis factor, interleukin-1, and granulocyte–macrophage colony-stimulating factor.

These mediators promote morphological changes such as the spreading and clumping seen in **50b**. Metabolic changes include stimulation of the oxidative burst pathway, an upregulation of inflammatory cytokine production, and an increased expression of cell surface receptors mediating adhesion, phagocytosis, and antigen presentation.

Other macrophage-derived cytokines, such as interleukin-1 and transforming growth factor, provide an autocrine negative feedback mechanism by downregulating many of these macrophage functions. Macrophage-derived chemotactic factors, including leukotriene B4 and the interleukin-8 chemokine family, recruit neutrophils to the site of infection, while other products attract monocytes and lymphocytes. Additional interactions between macrophage-derived cytokines and epithelial cells, endothelial cells, fibroblasts, and lymphocyte subpopulations further alter the inflammatory response.

51 The patient whose X-ray (**51**) is shown here had polio 30 years ago and was clinically stable until recently when he developed fatigue, joint pains, muscle weakness, swallowing difficulties, and dyspnoea.

i. What disorder does this patient have, and what are the underlying factors responsible for his breathing abnormality?

ii. How is sleep affected in this disorder?

iii. How is this disorder managed?

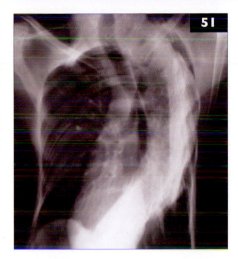

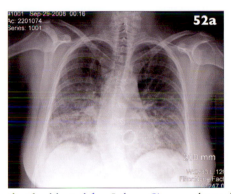

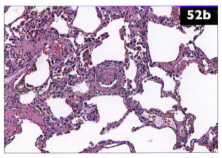

52 A 34-year-old female presented with shortness of breath and chest discomfort that had lasted for 5 days. Six months earlier, she had been intubated for a period of 12 days, had had slow resolution of her culture-negative pneumonia, suffered an upper extremity venous thrombosis in conjunction with a central line, was thrombocytopenic and given a diagnosis of idiopathic thrombocytopenic purpura, and was discharged on prednisone and warfarin, both of which were discontinued 2 weeks prior to her current presentation. She had suffered three miscarriages.

BAL returned pink fluid with a red blood cell count of 6400 cells/cm^3 and 165 white blood cells (68% mononuclear, 12% polymorphonuclear, 1% eosinophils). The anticardiolipin IgG was 69 IU and IgM was 22 IU (>20 IU being considered moderately positive). **52a** shows her chest X-ray, and **52b** a VATS biopsy.

i. What does the pathology show?

ii. What is the diagnosis?

51 i. This patient has post-polio syndrome, which usually occurs two to three decades after the acute infection and recovery. These patients usually have kyphoscoliosis, which causes restriction and can blunt the hypercapnic drive because of mechanical impairment. In addition, they may also have decreased respiratory drive as a result of damage to their medullary neurones and may also have respiratory muscle weakness. Patients who did not have respiratory involvement with the initial infection are unlikely to develop such weakness or kyphoscoliosis.

ii. In the early stages, respiration during sleep is more likely to be affected. Initially, short central apnoeas occur, and as the condition progresses these become longer and more frequent. Sleep abnormalities include decreased sleep efficiency and increased arousal frequency. Eventually, awake respiration can be affected.

iii. Patients with predominantly central sleep apnoea should be managed with BiPAP during sleep, which is delivered via a nasal mask. A 20 cmH_2O inspiratory pressure support can be achieved with this, with expiratory support of 5 cmH_2O delivering a defined number of breaths. This must be timed support, per minute rather than triggered by the patient's breathing. Some patients who have more severe disease that includes irregularities in awake breathing will require ventilatory support during both sleep and wakefulness. Early ventilation systems included the negative-pressure tank apparatus. Nasal positive-pressure ventilation is now more commonly used.

52 i. Alveolar hemorrhage and small-vessel thrombotic occlusion.

ii. Catastrophic antiphospholipid antibody syndrome. Pulmonary damage in this syndrome involves both chronic venous macro- and micro-thromboembolism, but non-thromboembolic lung injury caused by capillaritis with pulmonary haemorrhage is increasingly seen. The diagnosis of catastrophic antiphospholipid antibody syndrome requires:

1. Evidence of involvement of three or more organs, systems, or tissues.
2. Development of manifestations simultaneously or in less than 1 week.
3. Confirmation by histopathology of small-vessel occlusion in at least one organ or tissue.
4. Laboratory confirmation of the presence of antiphospholipid antibodies.

The diagnosis is considered definite if all four criteria are met and is probable with:

- All four criteria with only two organs, systems, or tissues.
- All four criteria without confirmation 6 weeks apart due to death.
- Criteria 1, 2, and 4.
- Criteria 1, 3, and 4 with a third event in more than a week but less than 1 month despite anticoagulation.

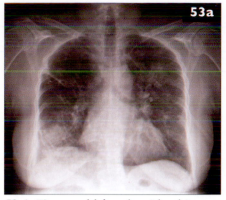

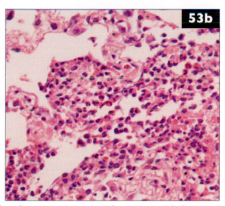

53 A 58-year-old female with a history of asthma presents with a 3-month history of dry cough, lower extremity oedema, fatigue, and shortness of breath that has worsened markedly over the last 2 weeks accompanied by a 9 kg (20 lb) weight gain. On physical examination, she has bibasilar crackles, her jugular venous pressure is elevated, and she has bilateral lower extremity oedema. Her chest X-ray is shown in **53a**.

She has a white blood cell count of 7000 cells/cm^3, 25% of which are eosinophils. BAL has demonstrated a white blood cell count of 133 cells/cm^3 with 4% neutrophils, 20% lymphocytes, 17% eosinophils, and 55% macrophages. Her transbronchial lung biopsy is shown in **53b**.
i. What does the lung biopsy show?
ii. What is the diagnosis?
iii. What is the treatment?

54 This 32-year-old male presented with a 3-month history of a dry cough with fevers and night sweats.
i. Describe the chest X-ray (**54**).
ii. What is the differential diagnosis?
iii. How might the diagnosis be made?

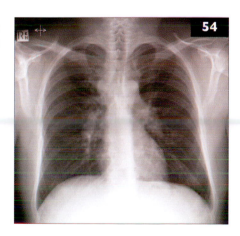

53 i. The lung biopsy shows diffuse inflammation with an infiltration of eosinophils.

ii. Chronic eosinophilic pneumonia. This results from an idiopathic accumulation of eosinophils in the lungs with inflammation and tissue destruction resulting from the release of eosinophilic granules. Patients generally present in the third or fourth decade, and the condition is more common in females. Symptoms may be present for months prior to diagnosis (a mean of 7.7 months in one study). Fifty per cent of patients have an associated history of asthma.

Establishing the diagnosis involves excluding other causes of pulmonary eosinophilia such as Churg–Strauss syndrome, drug- or toxin-induced pulmonary eosinophilia (non-steroidal anti-inflammatory agents, nitrofurantoin, ampicillin, aluminum silicate and particulate metal exposure, crack and heroine inhalation), helminthic infections, and tropical pulmonary eosinophilia. The chest X-ray classically shows the 'photographic negative shadow of pulmonary oedema', but this finding is only present in 25–50% of patients.

iii. Chronic eosinophilic pneumonia is extremely corticosteroid responsive such that symptoms rapidly decrease with prednisone doses of 40–60 mg/day, and after 2–4 weeks radiographic findings decrease by 50% or resolve completely. Unfortunately, chronic eosinophilic pneumonia can recur if corticosteroids are tapered too rapidly. Accordingly, treatment should be continued for at least 2–3 months, and the doses should then be tapered. In one study, 75% of patients required therapy for more than 1 year, with the average duration of treatment being 19 months. Some patients require lifelong treatment.

54 i. The chest X-ray shows lymphadenopathy in the right paratracheal and left hilar regions.

ii. The differential diagnosis lies between sarcoid, TB, and lymphoma.

iii. The history does not help to differentiate between these conditions so a tissue diagnosis is mandatory. Once lymphadenopathy of the cervical (which commonly co-exists with mediastinal nodes) and other peripheral nodes has been excluded by physical examination and ultrasound examination of the neck, bronchoscopy may be a reasonable first step as it has a high yield for the diagnosis of sarcoid and TB. Furthermore, transbronchial biopsies should also be taken of lung parenchyma, which can demonstrate non-caseating granulomas in up to 70% of patients with sarcoid and 50% of those with TB. Transbronchial needle aspiration of the mediastinal lymph nodes can also be performed during bronchoscopy, and the technique has more recently become aided by ultrasound guidance (EBUS) for higher yields. If bronchoscopic samples are negative, mediastinoscopy is necessary for a definitive diagnosis.

55 This male patient feels well but has a squamous cell carcinoma in his right upper lobe.
i. What does this test (**55**) show?
ii. Should it be routine in asymptomatic subjects with lung cancer?
iii. What is the differential diagnosis of the abnormality?

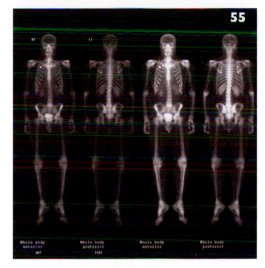

56 This is the chest X-ray (**56**) of a 54-year-old Bengali male who had haemoptysis when arriving at Heathrow airport to visit his family. On closer questioning, he gave a 3-month history of weight loss, malaise with night sweats, and a cough.
i. What is the likely diagnosis?
ii. How would you prove the diagnosis?
iii. In what circumstances would you need to take steps to assess the other passengers on the plane?

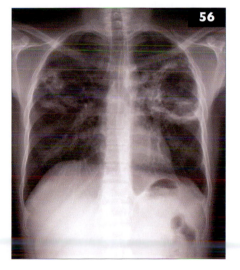

55 i. This isotope bone scan shows a single area of increased uptake in the anterior part of the right second rib, which, if malignant, would render the tumour inoperable.

ii. Routine bone scans in asymptomatic individuals are positive in 4–6% of cases. In half of these the cause will not be cancer, i.e. it will be a false-positive result. Any such lesion would therefore need to be confirmed by biopsy. This scan is therefore not recommended for routine staging.

iii. The differential diagnosis should also include Paget's disease, recent bone trauma, parathyroidism, and active arthritis.

A PET scan is more specific for identifying bony lesions due to malignancy, and when employed in potentially operable individuals, it makes bone scanning redundant. However, the bone scan remains useful in those with bone pains and lung cancer.

56 i. Active pulmonary TB.

ii. Sputum samples for microscopy for *Mycobacterium tuberculosis* using acid-fast or auramine staining. The presence of acid-fast bacilli (smear positive) is highly suggestive of TB, but can occur with disease resulting from environmental mycobacteria or some rare filamentous bacterial infection (e.g. *Nocardia*). Infection is confirmed by a positive culture, but even with modern fast culture techniques, this can take up to 6 weeks.

A positive culture also allows the identification of drug sensitivities, a vital consideration if resistance is suspected (e.g. in patients with poor compliance with previous treatment for TB, those who have received suboptimal treatment for other reasons, and those who have acquired the disease in countries with a high incidence of drug resistance, such as the Baltic States).

If the sputum is smear negative (no acid-fast bacilli present), the diagnosis may have to be clinical. Inflammatory markers such as CRP and ESR are usually high, but a positive tuberculin skin test or gamma-interferon test is to be expected in patients from countries with a high incidence of TB such as the Indian subcontinent, owing to frequent past exposure to *M. tuberculosis*; this is therefore of limited help in confirming the diagnosis. In many smear-negative patients, bronchoscopy to obtain bronchial washings from the affected area will be smear positive and can confirm the diagnosis.

iii. If the patient is smear positive, this indicates that there is a high bacillary load in the sputum ($>10^3$ bacteria/ml) and that close contacts are at risk of contracting the disease. Screening is usually limited to the immediate family and housemates. If, however, a smear-positive patient has recently flown on a flight of 8 hr or more duration, the passengers are advised to seek medical advice (World Health Organization, *Tuberculosis and Air Travel: Guidelines for Prevention and Control*, 2nd edition, 2006).

57 This chest radiograph (57) is of a 26-year-old male who had repeated syncopal episodes and required permanent pacemaker insertion for complete heart block. He had also experienced several months of lethargy and intermittent dull retrosternal chest pain.
i. What diagnostic possibility does the radiography suggest?
ii. What investigations could be undertaken?
iii. What is the cause of the pain?
iv. When are corticosteroids indicated?

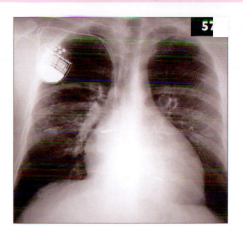

58 This chest radiograph (58) is of a patient with cystic fibrosis.
i. What does it show?
ii. Why is a spontaneous pneumothorax different in cystic fibrosis?
iii. What is the optimum medical management?
iv. What is the optimum surgical management?

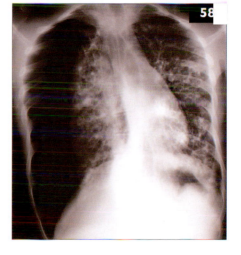

57 i. This patient has stage III sarcoidosis with cardiac involvement. Cardiac disease in this condition may cause a range of ventricular and supraventricular arrhythmias and conduction defects. Cardiomyopathy may rarely develop.

ii. ECG and Holter monitoring to document arrhythmias; two-dimensional echocardiography may show ventricular septal thinning, localized regional wall abnormalities, or a generalized cardiomyopathy. Thallium scintigraphy may show regions of abnormal perfusion. Endocardial biopsy may yield positive histology in less than 40% of cases. Cardiac MRI is useful for identifying potential cardiac sarcoidosis.

iii. Chest pain is common in sarcoidosis (at least 25%) and may be pleuritic or dull and retrosternal. It may be severe and sometimes mimic a myocardial infarct. Cardiac sarcoidosis is a difficult diagnosis to establish without a myocardial biopsy. Even then, a clear association between an arrhythmia and sarcoidosis is difficult unless the sarcoidosis is clearly active in other sites.

iv. Arrhythmias and cardiomyopathy should be treated in the usual way. Corticosteroids would be indicated if standard treatment were ineffective or if the sarcoidosis were active at other sites. Monitoring of the response of cardiac sarcoid to corticosteroids is difficult.

58 i. A large right tension pneumothorax. The incidence of pneumothorax increases with disease severity and may be associated with a poor prognosis. It occurs due to the rupture of subpleural blebs through the visceral pleura, usually in the upper lobes. The incidence of pneumothorax is higher in patients with widespread pre-existing lung disease.

ii. A pneumothorax in cystic fibrosis is different from that occurring in other patients owing to its association with large amounts of purulent secretions. This can make physiotherapy difficult and lung re-expansion very slow. In addition, patients with cystic fibrosis who get pneumothoraces usually have severe disease and can become extremely sick with a pneumothorax.

iii. Patients with pneumothoraces need prompt medical treatment. At the time of the pneumothorax, they should be commenced on intravenous antibiotics. If large, the pneumothorax should be drained immediately. If the patient is breathless, a small pneumothorax requires intercostal drainage under radiological control. An intubated pneumothorax makes physiotherapy easier. A small pneumothorax in an asymptomatic patient may be aspirated or observed for 2–3 days.

iv. If a pneumothorax fails to resolve with maximal medical management within a week, prompt surgical intervention should be considered. With the advent of organ transplantation, extensive pleurodesis or pleurectomy is not appropriate. The best surgical option is video-assisted stapling of the apical subpleural bleb under direct vision.

	Result	Normal range
PEFR (l/min)	450	383–518
FEV_1 (l)	2.75	2.34–3.16
FVC (l)	4.05	3.45–4.66
FEV_1/FVC (%)	69	58–79
DL_{CO} (haemoglobin corrected)	7.88	6.70–9.06
Alveolar volume (l)	1.47	1.25–1.69
K_{CO} (haemoglobin corrected)	5.36	2.63–3.55

K_{CO} = transfer coefficient in DL_{CO}/alveolar volume.

59 A 30-year-old male was admitted with fever, cough with haemoptysis, and dyspnoea. A few red blood cells but no microorganisms were noted on a sputum Gram stain.
i. What does the lung function test (*Table*) show?
ii. What does this chest radiograph (**59**) show?
iii. What is the cause?
iv. Name three important conditions associated with this and the laboratory investigations that would differentiate them.

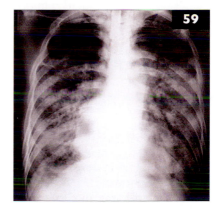

60 This is a radiological imaging test (**60**) of a 40-year-old male presenting with dyspnoea on exertion that had evolved over a week and was not associated with fevers, cough or any respiratory signs. His ECG showed a sinus tachycardia, right bundle branch block, and inverted T waves in leads V1–V3.
i. What is this investigation, and what does it show?
ii. How should the patient be managed?
iii. How else may this patient's condition present?

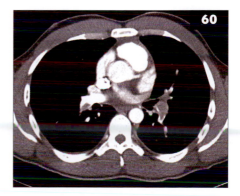

59 i. A high K_{CO}, i.e. increased diffusion capacity across the alveolar–capillary membrane. Additional carbon monoxide uptake occurs in the lungs because of the presence of alveolar haemorrhage.

ii. A bilateral alveolar filling pattern.

iii. Pulmonary haemorrhage.

iv. Three important associated conditions and the laboratory investigations that differentiate them are:

• Goodpasture's disease: antiglomerular basement membrane antibody.

• Wegener's granulomatosis: cytoplasmic ANCA.

• Systemic vasculitis: antinuclear antibody, anti-double-stranded DNA antibody.

60 i. This is a CT pulmonary angiogram, and it confirms the clinical suspicion of pulmonary embolus. There are filling defects in both pulmonary arteries due to the presence of a clot. CT pulmonary angiograms have transformed the diagnosis of pulmonary emboli by providing a rapid test that is readily available for emergencies and can be used in patients with other significant lung pathology, whereas clinicians previously had to rely on *V/Q* scans, which are not readily interpretable in the presence of other lung disease such as COPD.

ii. As well as fluid resuscitation and oxygen, the patient needs to be anticoagulated with treatment-dose heparin or low molecular weight heparin for several days and then to take warfarin to prevent recurrence. How long warfarin should be taken depends on the clinical situation: if the patient has a well-documented predisposing factor for a pulmonary embolus, such as a recent operation or long-haul flight, the warfarin can probably be discontinued after 3 months. However, if there is no risk factor, warfarin is conventionally suggested for a longer period, usually 6 months. If this is a second episode, a procoagulant screen will be necessary, and consideration will be given to lifelong treatment with warfarin. Whether investigations for occult malignancy should be performed is controversial as the detection rate is less than 5%.

iii. Pulmonary emboli can present, like this case, as a cause of acute dyspnoea and may be associated with haemoptysis and pleuritic chest pain. On examination, there are often few signs, but there may be a pleural rub or small effusion. Massive pulmonary emboli can present with cardiogenic shock, signs of right heart strain, and sometimes cardiac arrest. Multiple small pulmonary emboli can cause pulmonary hypertension and present with an insidious onset of dyspnoea; there may also be signs of pulmonary hypertension on examination.

61 A 65-year-old ex-smoker with a past history of TB as a child and of laryngeal carcinoma necessitating a laryngectomy at age 61 presented having coughed up approximately 150 ml of fresh blood. He had been previously well except for a history of minor haemoptysis over several months.

i. What are the common causes of a major life-threatening haemoptysis, and what are the most likely potential causes in this patient?

ii. What is the immediate management of this patient?

iii. How can further major haemoptysis be prevented?

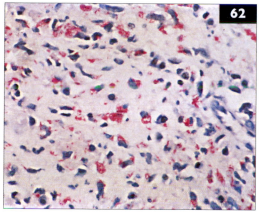

62 This histology (**62**) was obtained from a mediastinal lymph node of an HIV-positive male. What stain has been used, and what does it show?

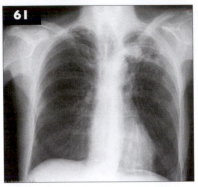

61 i. The common causes of major haemoptysis (>200 ml blood over 24 hr) are bronchiectasis, lung cancer, and mycetomas. Rarer causes include TB, invasive aspergillosis, PAVM, a pulmonary artery aneurysm, a vascular–bronchial fistula, and vasculitis. Other common causes of haemoptysis, e.g. pneumonia, pulmonary embolism, and left ventricular failure, generally cause only minor haemoptysis.

In this patient, the history of laryngeal carcinoma means that he is at high risk of developing a lung carcinoma, and the previous TB could have caused focal bronchiectasis or lung cavities that have subsequently been colonized by *Aspergillus* to form a mycetoma. The chest radiograph (**61**) demonstrates bilateral apical scarring and fibrosis with loss of volume in the upper lobes and a cavity in the left upper lobe, but no obvious lung malignancy. The cavity does not contain an obvious mycetoma.
ii. The immediate management includes obtaining a full blood count, clotting, and cross-match. It is rare for a patient to lose enough blood to require transfusion, but if this is the case, the patient is at high risk and active measures will be necessary to try to stop the bleeding (see below). A chest X-ray may identify the likely source, but CT scanning is often necessary to identify patches of bronchiectasis or confirm potential cancers or mycetomas identified on the chest X-ray. Bronchoscopy is helpful in identifying the side from which the bleeding is originating and can give helpful diagnostic information if bronchial washings are positive for *Aspergillus* or the cytology identifies fungal elements or malignant cells. Patients are often given antibiotics in case bacterial infection has helped to cause the bleeding (although there is little evidence that they are beneficial), and the pro-thrombotic agent tranexamic acid can be used.
iii. Life-threatening haemoptysis or continuing major haemoptysis needs intervention with either surgery to remove the affected lobe, or arterial embolization. Embolization is often the only option due to the patient's poor lung function or underlying condition, and also because there are often extensive scarring and pleural changes that make surgery technically challenging. Antifungal agents (eg itraconazole 200 mg twice a day) may help in patients with major haemoptysis caused by mycetomas.

62 A Ziehl–Neelsen stain has been used, with which acid-fast bacilli appear red. This should be distinguished from the more rapid auramine fluorescence stain with which acid-fast bacilli fluoresce on a dark background. Neither stain is specific for *Mycobacterium tuberculosis* and may identify other non-tuberculous mycobacteria, including the *Mycobacterium avium* complex.

63 i. What is the mechanism of action of CPAP (**63**) in OSA?

ii. What are the potential side-effects of nasal CPAP?

iii. How compliant are patients with OSA who are prescribed CPAP?

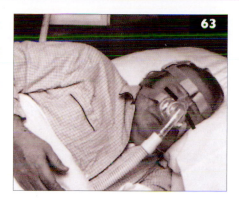

64 i. Describe the appearances in this chest radiograph (**64**).

ii. What are the likely causative organisms?

iii. What are the causes of a swollen lobe in the presence of pneumonia?

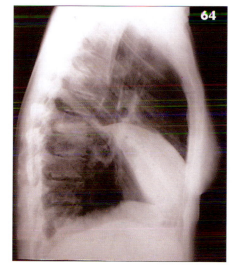

63 i. CPAP acts as a pneumatic splint. It increases the intraluminal pressure within the upper airway and thus counteracts the transmural forces that favour airway closure. The typical site of obstruction in patients with OSA is between the nasopharynx and the larynx. This region is narrowed during sleep due to a reduction in muscle tone, and individuals with OSA have on average a smaller diameter pharyngeal lumen.

ii. Poorly fitting masks result in air leakage. This not only reduces the applied airway pressure, but also can cause conjunctivitis if the air leak is directed towards the eye. A poorly fitting mask can also bruise or cause ulceration of the bridge of the nose. These problems can be avoided by selecting and properly fitting the appropriate mask type and size. Most patients initially experience nasal congestion, but this complaint frequently diminishes with continued use. Intranasal vasoconstrictors, anticholinergic agents, and steroids have been used in this setting. Humidification of air within the CPAP system can also help if these measures are ineffective.

iii. Compliance rates vary from 45% to 80% and studies show the average hours used is fewer than 5 per night. There are no consistent clinical predictors of compliance, although one study suggested that patients who complain of side-effects were those found to be less compliant. Follow-up and support by physicians, as well as personalizing the type of CPAP device and mask, may be important in improving patient compliance.

64 i. This lateral chest radiograph (**64**) shows homogeneous consolidation within the middle lobe. The horizontal fissure is bowed upwards, suggesting some swelling of the lobe.

ii. *Streptococcus pneumoniae* is the most common cause of CAP and is the most typical cause of lobar pneumonia. However, it is often unappreciated that most other common bacterial causes of pneumonia can also cause lobar consolidation, including *Legionella*, and *Staphylococcus aureus*, and as many as 50% of *Mycoplasma pneumoniae* pneumonias are lobar.

iii. *Klebsiella pneumoniae* is also a cause of a swollen lobe on the chest radiograph but as in this example, which is due to *Mycoplasma pneumoniae*, any bacterial pathogen can potentially do this.

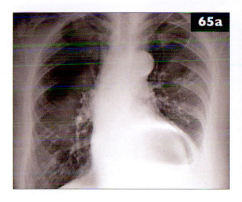

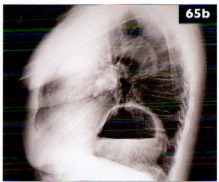

65 The chest radiographs (**65a**, **65b**) and barium swallow (**65c**) belong to a 68-year-old female.

i. What lesion is demonstrated?

ii. What symptoms is the patient likely to complain of?

iii. Which form of management is likely to be advised, and why would it be recommended?

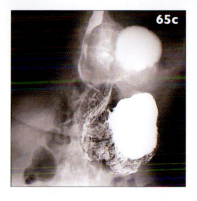

66 i. What is the likely cell type of this lung cancer (**66**) and why?

ii. How is it staged?

iii. What is the optimal treatment for 'limited disease' presentations?

iv. What are the 2- and 5-year survival rates after treatment?

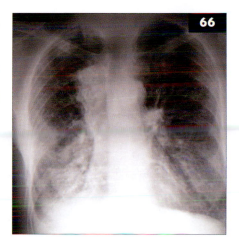

65 i. A 'rolling' hiatus hernia. In this condition, the herniated stomach protrudes into the chest through the hiatus beside the lower oesophagus. The oesophagogastric junction is usually normally located.

ii. These patients may be remarkably symptom-free, and the condition may be spotted as an incidental finding. Moderate dysphagia and fullness with meals are, however, common and may worsen as a meal progresses due to distension of the intrathoracic stomach. Acid reflux is not a feature because the oesophagogastric junction is usually competent and because the intrathoracic stomach further prevents reflux by pressing on the lower oesophagus.

iii. Surgical management is usually advised. This is the only effective way to manage dysphagia due to this condition, and if the hernia is not reduced there is a risk of ulceration and perforation or even strangulation of the herniated stomach.

Reduction of the hernia may be accomplished via a low left lateral thoracotomy or a laparotomy. Advantages of a thoracic approach include better access to the oesophagogastric junction and hernial sac. An abdominal approach may be helpful in the event that concurrent abdominal surgery is required but offers poorer access to divide the adhesions, which are frequently present in the hernial sac.

66 i. This is likely to be a small-cell cancer because the disease appears very bulky. This most aggressive cell type classically presents with advanced spread within the chest to the hilar and mediastinal lymph nodes, the primary tumour often being indistinguishable from the nodal disease. Pleural effusion is present in 20% of presentations.

ii. This type of cancer is staged as limited disease, which is confined to the hemithorax and ipsilateral supraclavicular fossa, or extensive disease, which is present when disease is also found outside the hemithorax. The recommended staging tests include routine blood tests, chest X-ray and CT scanning of the thorax to include the liver and adrenal glands. Bone and brain scans are made only if symptoms indicate.

iii. Treatment is by cytotoxic chemotherapy. Cisplatin and etoposide form the drug combination of choice for four or six courses. Around 50% of patients will obtain a complete response and another 30% a partial response. Those with a complete response and a good partial response should receive mediastinal radiotherapy, which confers a 5% better 2-year survival, and also prophylactic whole-brain radiotherapy. There is no agreed effective second-line therapy, although reasonable results have been reported with oral topotecan.

iv. The overall 2-year survival for small-cell carcinoma is 7%. For those with a good prognosis (high performance status and normal biochemistry), the 2-year survival is 15–20%. Of those alive at 2 years, 25% will relapse with small-cell disease, and another 20% will develop non-small-cell lung cancers within 5 years.

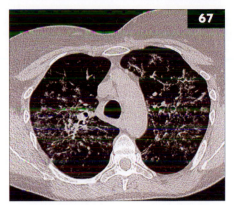

67 A 45-year-old female, originally from Jamaica, has a 3-year history of a dry cough and gradual exertional breathlessness. Her HRCT is shown here (**67**).
i. Describe the HRCT appearances.
ii. How may the diagnosis be confirmed?
iii. When is treatment indicated?

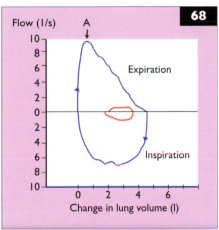

68 This 45-year-old, non-smoking male produced the flow–volume curve in **68**.
i. Is it of normal or abnormal shape?
ii. What is point A? How is it usually measured?
iii. Why does the expiratory curve decrease progressively in flow as the RV is approached?
iv. Why is the inspiratory curve semicircular in shape and dissimilar to the expiratory curve?

67 i. The HRCT axial cut demonstrates lung parenchymal nodules in a bronchovascular distribution, characteristic of sarcoidosis.

ii. The diagnosis may be confirmed pathologically by the demonstration of non-caseating granulomas and a negative culture for TB. This may be achieved by transbronchial or open lung biopsy, the sampling of enlarged mediastinal nodes, or the biopsy of involved extrathoracic sites.

iii. Oral corticosteroid treatment should be considered in patients with severe, persistent, or progressively worsening respiratory symptoms that interfere with daily life. Treatment should also be instituted if lung function progressively deteriorates over 6 months. A fall in VC of 10–15% and/or transfer factor for carbon monoxide of >20%, confirmed on more than one occasion, is considered significant. Treatment should not be commenced in asymptomatic patients in the absence of other organ involvement.

68 i. This is a normal-shaped curve.

ii. The expiratory limb is triangular in shape. Following a full inspiration, the lung's recoil pressure is maximal, as is the pleural pressure, because the thoracic muscles are stretched to provide maximal expiratory force. The onset of expiratory flow is explosive and reaches its peak rate within 0.01 s, i.e. at point A. This is the PEFR and is usually measured with a peak flow meter.

iii. The expiratory curve decreases its flow gradually as the lung volume drops from TLC to RV. This graded decline reflects the gradual drop in the lung's elastic recoil as the lung gets smaller, as well as the gradual reduction in airway calibre during expiration; also, muscular force on the lung (pleural pressure) slowly decreases as the thoracic cage changes position during expiration and the respiratory muscles shorten.

iv. Inspiration does not reach an instant maximal flow, in contrast to expiration, which does so owing to the inspiratory recruitment of dynamic forces. On expiration, the respiratory muscles contract, and the power increases almost instantly from the start of expiration to achieve a maximal flow within milliseconds. This process takes much longer at the start of inspiration as the muscle forces that generate flow take longer to develop, and maximal inspiratory flow is only achieved by the midpoint of the inspiratory VC. It then slows again as the maximum inspired volume is reached as a consequence of muscular contraction slowing at the higher lung volumes (TLC). This causes the semicircular appearance of the inspiratory flow–volume curve.

69 i. What is this, and how does it work?
ii. What are the indications for its use?
iii. What is the optimum length of time per day it should be used for?

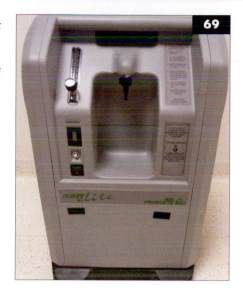

70 This female of 58 has had similar appearances on her chest radiograph (70) for over 5 years. She does not have significant respiratory symptoms. What is the differential diagnosis?

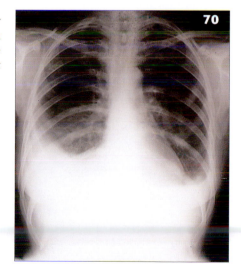

> **Criteria for long-term oxygen therapy**
> $FEV_1 < 1.5$ l
> *and*
> PaO_2 less than 7.3 kPa when stable*
> *or*
> PaO_2 greater than 7.3 kPa and less than 8 kPa when stable,* as well as one of:
> • Secondary polycythaemia
> • Nocturnal hypoxaemia (SaO_2 less than 90% for more than 30% of the time)
> • Peripheral oedema
> • Pulmonary hypertension
> *Measurement of arterial blood gases on two occasions at least 3 weeks apart in patients who have a definitive diagnosis of COPD and who are receiving optimum medical management

69 i. An oxygen concentrator. Room air is entrained into the machine, and nitrogen is adsorbed by zeolite material, resulting in high-concentration oxygen. Concentrators are typically able to deliver concentrations between 50% and 95% at a flow rate of up to 5 l/min. Long-term oxygen therapy should be prescribed for patients in respiratory failure (defined as a PaO_2 <8 kPa).
ii. The specific criteria for long-term oxygen therapy in patients with COPD are summarised in the *Box*.
iii. In patients who qualify for long-term oxygen therapy, oxygen should be prescribed for at least 15 hr/day, although survival may be augmented when used for more than 20 hr/day.

70 The chest radiograph shows moderate bilateral pleural effusions. The absence of cardiac enlargement and significant dyspnoea should exclude left ventricular failure, although cardiac failure can occur with a normal cardiac silhouette in patients with mitral stenosis or constrictive pericarditis. It is most likely that the patient has an inflammatory pleurisy, probably due to autoimmune disease such as systemic lupus erythematosus or rheumatoid arthritis. The patient shown here suffered from chronic rheumatoid arthritis. Other possible causes include vasculitides such as polyarteritis nodosa, Wegener's granulomatosis and polyserositis, drug reactions, e.g. hydralazine, phenytoin, phenothiazines, and practolol, lymphatic hypoplasia (yellow nail syndrome) and hypothyroidism. In general, bilateral effusions suggest a systemic cause and unilateral fluid a local cause.

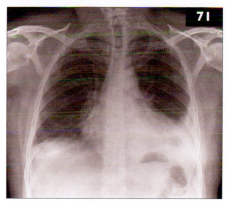

71 This patient presented with cough and fever and was diagnosed as having a CAP.
i. What complication of CAP does the chest X-ray (**71**) show?
ii. How should this case be managed?

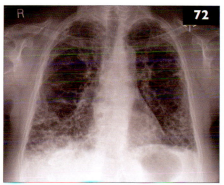

72 This is the chest radiograph (**72**) of a 66-year-old Middle Eastern female presenting with a constant cough productive of purulent sputum up to one cupful per day.
i. What is the likely diagnosis, and how can this be proved?
ii. What are the causes of this disease?
iii. What investigations are needed, and what may the sputum contain?

71 i. The chest X-ray shows left basal consolidation with an associated pleural effusion.

ii. Although most effusions associated with CAP are simple parapneumonic effusions that will resolve without intervention, significant pleural effusions should be tapped to exclude an complicated parapneumonic effusion (defined as pleural fluid pH <7.2, lactase dehydrogenase >1000 IU/l or glucose <2.2 mmol/l) or empyema (visibly turbid fluid or a positive Gram stain or culture for bacteria). If these are present, the fluid should be drained. Persisting fever or blood tests showing high inflammatory markers or a raised platelet or white cell count would be a further indication that the fluid should be drained to exclude pleural infection as a cause for the failure of the patient to improve.

72 i. The history is suggestive of severe bronchiectasis, and the chest radiograph shows a large number of ring shadows suggestive of dilated, thick-walled bronchi, compatible with this diagnosis. Bronchiectasis can be confirmed by HRCT scans of the lungs, which will show dilated bronchi (>110% of the diameter of the accompanying artery) that are thick walled. There may be 'tree-in-bud' changes, especially during active disease, due to mucous filling the small airways.

ii. There are a large number of causes of bronchiectasis, although in industrialized nations most cases are idiopathic. Worldwide, the most common cause is severe childhood infection (e.g. whooping cough, measles, pneumonia, TB). Other important causes are cystic fibrosis, primary ciliary dyskinesia, immunoglobulin deficiency, focal bronchial obstruction, atypical mycobacterial infection (especially *Mycobacterium avium-intracellulare*), and allergic bronchopulmonary aspergillosis. Bronchiectasis has recently been increasing recognized in patients with severe COPD, being present on CT scans in 25% of these patients, and in long-term survivors with HIV infection.

iii. The patient will need an HRCT of the thorax, lung function testing (bronchiectasis is associated with asthma or fixed small airways obstruction that can be severe), total IgG and IgE levels, *Aspergillus* antibodies and skin testing, as well as sputum culture for bacteria, fungi (to look for *Aspergillus*), and mycobacteria (to exclude atypical mycobacterial infection that can both cause and complicate cases of bronchiectasis). The bacteria present in bronchiectasis include *Streptococcus pneumoniae*, *Haemophilus influenzae*, *Moraxella catarrhalis* and *Staphylococcus aureus* (especially in cystic fibrosis). In severe bronchiectasis, patients almost invariably become colonized with *Pseudomonas aeruginosa* and can acquire more unusual environmental bacteria such as *Burkholderia cepacia* and *Stenotrophomonas*.

73 This is the chest radiograph (**73**) of a teenager who has had a lifetime history of cough productive of frequently purulent sputum and needs enzyme supplementation of her diet to prevent malabsorption.
i. What is the condition?
ii. How is it inherited, and what is the genetic defect?
iii. How is the diagnosis confirmed?
iv. What are the main respiratory complications, and which pathogens are likely to be isolated from her sputum?

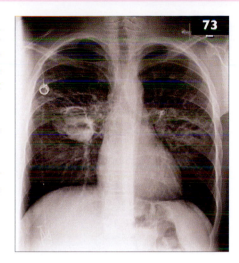

74 This scan (**74**) was taken 5 years after the patient, a 55-year-old man, presented with a blood-stained pleural effusion. At that time examination of the fluid and bronchoscopy were negative. What is the abnormality shown, and what are the possible causes?

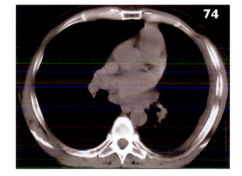

73 i. Cystic fibrosis leading to bronchiectasis and impaired exocrine (and in some patients endocrine) pancreatic function requiring pancreatic enzyme supplementation. The basic pathophysiology is excessively thick mucous production, leading to a failure to clear bacterial infection from the lungs, airway inflammation, and blockage of the pancreatic ducts.

ii. This is an autosomal recessive gene defect affecting the CFTR protein, an ATP-binding cassette (ABC) transporter ion channel in epithelial cell membranes. A very large number (>1400) of different mutations have been described, but the most common in Western populations is the deletion of phenylalanine at position 508 (F508Δ), which is present in approximately 66% of cases. Most cases of cystic fibrosis result in fatal disease, although with improved medical care, the median age of death has risen to 37 years. Exactly how impaired function of the CFTR leads to an inability to clear respiratory secretions and chronic bronchial infection is not, however, clear.

iii. The diagnosis is confirmed by an elevated sweat chloride level (>60 mmol/l) on a sweat test. In patients with equivocal results (30–60 mmol/l), nasal potential difference can be used, but this is a technically difficult test. CFTR genotyping will help as long as the patient has one of the 50 or so more common mutations, which are responsible for 80–90% of cases.

iv. Cystic fibrosis causes severe, mainly upper lobe bronchiectasis (in contrast to non-cystic fibrosis bronchiectiasis, which tends to affect the lower or middle lobes) with a distal progressive small airways obstruction, resulting in respiratory failure, cor pulmonale, and death. Haemoptysis and pneumothorax are common complications, and patients can be colonized with *Aspergillus* and develop allergic bronchopulmonary aspergillosis or semi-invasive chronic necrotizing aspergillosis.

The common pathogens are *Staphylococcus aureus* (which is relatively rare in non-cystic fibrosis bronchectasis) *Haemophilus influenzae*, *Moraxella catarrhalis*, and *Streptococcus pneumoniae* in early disease, but most patients are eventually colonized with *Pseudomonas aeruginosa*. Severely affected patients can also be colonized with *Burkholderia cepacia*, which can be associated with a rapid deterioration in lung function (the 'cepacia syndrome'). Recently, *Streptococcus milleri* species have been identified as common pathogens in patients with cystic fibrosis, and they can also develop superinfection with non-tuberculous mycobacteria.

74 Benign pleural thickening. In contrast to the scan of malignant pleural mesothelioma, the pleural thickening is smooth and diffuse, with only slight constriction of the hemithorax. A blood-stained pleural effusion is always suggestive of malignancy, but the long history makes this unlikely and this case was, in fact, due to benign asbestos-related pleurisy.

75 A 65-year-old male is a smoker and has a history of seropositive rheumatoid arthritis. Following a short history of cough, a chest X-ray (**75**) was performed.
i. Describe the image.
ii. What are the possible causes of the lesions?
iii. What investigations would you perform?

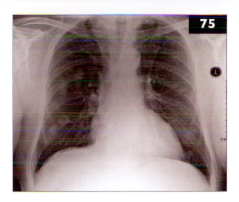

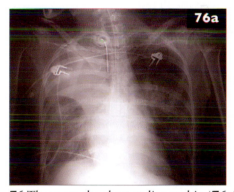

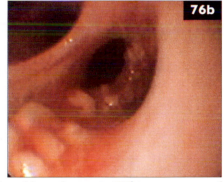

76 These are the chest radiographic (**76a**) and bronchoscopic (**76b**) appearance of a 24-year-old female in whom systemic lupus erythematosus had been diagnosed 6 months earlier. Her initial joint symptoms and rash had been successfully controlled on steroids, but 4 weeks before admission to ICU she developed symptoms suggestive of cerebral involvement, and the steroid dose was increased. She was admitted with respiratory distress, circulatory collapse, and disseminated intravascular coagulation. Gram-negative sepsis was confirmed, and she improved with antibiotic and standard supportive therapy. Pulsed cyclophosphamide was subsequently started for lupus cerebritis diagnosed on MRI scanning. Several weeks later, she suffered a massive haemoptysis, and the chest radiograph and bronchoscopy were performed at this time. Lesions similar to those pictured were present throughout the bronchial tree.
i. Describe the bronchoscopic appearances.
ii. Which organism is likely to be responsible for the respiratory problems?

75 i. The chest X-ray shows multiple 1–2 cm soft tissue nodules in both lungs, one of which is clearly peripheral in the left apex, with a further lesion in the right lower lobe. These lesions are cavitating, as seen in the right lower lobe.

ii. Possible causes of each lesion include malignancy, rheumatoid nodules, and infection.

iii. A CT/PET scan may differentiate malignancy from other causes. However, infection and rheumatoid nodules may also exhibit low-grade uptake on a PET scan. Rheumatoid lesions are always peripheral on the radiograph, may cavitate, and are seldom more than 1.5 cm in diameter. If there is doubt concerning the aetiology, a biopsy is recommended, particularly if the PET scan is positive.

76 i. The chest radiograph (**76a**) shows a densely consolidated right upper lobe with infiltrates in the middle and lower lobes. The bronchoscopy (**76b**) shows mucosal infiltration with white, nodular lesions, suggestive of a fungal infection.

ii. Histology of the bronchial biopsies showed extensive infiltration with fungal hyphae but minimal inflammatory infiltrate. *Aspergillus fumigatus* was subsequently isolated. The diagnosis is invasive aspergillosis, an important complication in immunocompromised patients. It usually presents as a necrotizing cavitating pneumonia unresponsive to standard antibiotics. The pulmonary features in this case are rare, but a wide variety of presentations have been described. Diagnosis may be difficult, with both sputum culture and serology frequently being negative. Biopsy specimens are usually required to make the diagnosis. Extrapulmonary dissemination to the liver, kidney, gastrointestinal tract, and brain occurs in about 25% of cases.

Treatment was with intravenous liposomal and nebulized amphotericin followed by oral itraconazole. The patient recovered, and a follow-up chest radiograph at 3 months was normal.

Aspergillus species can affect the lungs in several ways:
• Allergic bronchopulmonary aspergillosis in asthma.
• Aspergilloma, i.e. a fungus ball infects pre-existing cavities.
• Chronic necrotizing pulmonary aspergillosis.
• *Aspergillus* tracheobronchitis.
• Invasive aspergillosis, as in this case.
The last two develop in immunocompromised hosts.

77 i. What is this (77)?
ii. For which patients may it be prescribed?
iii. What are the benefits of the treatment, and how long does treatment last?

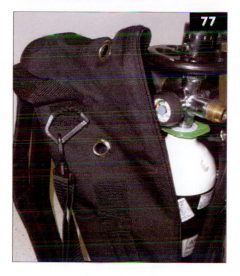

78 A 45-year-old female has a 5-year history of asthma. She has been well controlled on low doses of inhaled corticosteroids. Over the last 4 months, she has noticed that she has required the use of her short-acting bronchodilator several times per week, has awoken at night due to coughing, and has had two exacerbations of her asthma requiring oral steroids. How would you manage her case?

79 i. What is the abnormality here (79)?
ii. How do you know which lobe is affected?
iii. What are the likely causes?

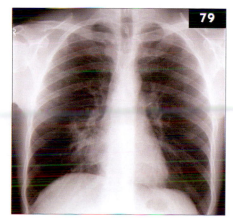

77 i. This is a portable oxygen cylinder.

ii. It allows patients with severe COPD or other lung disease to maintain exercise. People already on long-term oxygen therapy who wish to continue their oxygen therapy outside the home should have ambulatory oxygen provided. Ambulatory oxygen is also commonly prescribed in the context of short-burst oxygen therapy for patients who have documented exercise desaturation and improvement with oxygen therapy to maintain saturations above 90%.

iii. Despite the high cost of short-burst oxygen, there is very limited evidence to support its use. Various products are available. Oxygen cylinders may contain compressed gas or liquid oxygen and may be used with an oxygen-conserving device. When used at 2 l/min, a small oxygen cylinder that can be carried by the patient will last approximately 90 min. An oxygen-conserving device (allowing flow only during inspiration) can prolong this up to 4 hr.

78 This lady has symptoms suggesting that her asthma is uncontrolled. The first steps would be to ensure adherence to her inhaled corticosteroids and to check her inhaler technique. A careful history, enquiring about new allergen exposure, e.g. a new pet, is important. She is currently at step 2 of the GINA/BTS guidelines for asthma management (see Question 1). Once other potential causes of her worsening symptoms have been excluded, her pharmacological management should be stepped up. Step 3 of the GINA/BTS guidelines favours adding a long-acting beta-agonist, e.g. salmeterol or formoterol, to her current regime. This is most commonly done by switching to a combination of steroid + long-acting beta-agonist inhaler. This strategy has been shown to be more effective than just increasing the dose of the inhaled steroids alone.

79 i. The chest X-ray is of a collapsed right middle lobe.

ii. Middle lobe collapse causes the right border of the heart to be obscured. Unlike in lower lobe collapse, the diaphragmatic contour is preserved. As the lobe is relatively small, collapse does not result in mediastinal deviation.

iii. The common causes are lobar pneumonia, a lung tumour with occlusion of the middle lobe orifice, and post-tuberculous occlusion of the middle lobe airway as old TB glands at the hilum from a primary infection cause external compression (Brock's syndrome). A slow-growing benign tumour, e.g. carcinoid, can occasionally cause the recurrent collapse of an airway, which will become permanent in time.

80 Sand-blasting carries an occupational hazard.
i. Which pneumoconiosis is associated with this occupational exposure?
ii. What other occupations pose similar risks?

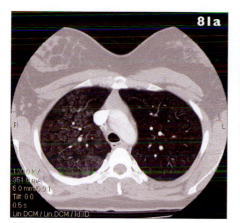

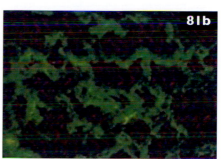

81 A 20-year-old female presented with 1-week of haemoptysis and shortness of breath. She had a three pack–year history of smoking a hookah nightly at a Middle Eastern restaurant. Physical examination revealed bilateral inspiratory crackles. Her chest CT is shown in 81a. Sequential BALs were increasingly bloody (72,000 cells/cm^3, 181,000 cells/cm^3, and 540,000 cells/cm^3, respectively). All serologies were negative, including ANCA, antinuclear antibodies, rheumatoid factor, antiglomerular basement membrane antibodies, scleroderma, and cryoglobulin. The patient's lung biopsy is shown in 81b.
i. What does the lung biopsy show?
ii. What is the diagnosis?
iii. Is it related to smoking?

80 i. Silicosis is a chronic, fibronodular interstitial lung disease caused by the inhalation of free crystalline silica (SiO_2). Silica occurs both complexed with other elements and in isolation as a 'free' form. The latter, occurring primarily as quartz, tridymite, and cristobalite, is associated with fibrotic lung disease. Tridymite and cristobalite are more fibrogenic than quartz.

ii. Sand-blasting is widely used to clean and etch stone and metal surfaces. Highly pressurized air or water drives a stream of abrasive sand into the workpiece. Very high concentrations of respirable silica are present in the resulting dust cloud. Non-siliceous particulates are increasingly used to minimize this risk, but if the target surface (e.g. stone) contains silica, significant exposure may still occur. Because silica is a major constituent of the earth's crust, mining, tunnelling, quarrying, and stone cutting may also entail significant exposure to silica-containing dust. Finely powdered quartz, known as silica flour or tripoli, is another common source of exposure as it is used as a polishing agent, as a dry lubricant in the rubber industry, and as a thickening agent in paints and plastics.

81 i. The lung biopsy shows areas of linear antibody deposition.

ii. Goodpasture's syndrome. Goodpasture's syndrome results from autoantibodies directed against the non-collagenous domain of the alpha-3 chain of type IV collagen on the alveolar and glomerular basement membranes, leading to alveolar haemorrhage and/or nephritis. Approximately 50% of patients present with nephritis alone, 45% present with nephritis and alveolar haemorrhage, and 5% present with alveolar haemorrhage alone (although in these, renal involvement may be seen on biopsy). In a small series, four of 10 patients with Goodpasture's localized to the lung subsequently developed renal dysfunction.

As many as 40% of patients with Goodpasture's syndrome may be seronegative for anti-basement membrane antibodies at the time of presentation. This phenomenon is attributed to the insensitivity of the ELISA assay for very low levels of circulating antibody (as the bulk of the antibody is deposited on the basement membranes). In some patients, circulating antibodies can be detected with a novel, highly sensitive biosensor assay system. Patients who are seronegative at presentation may become seropositive later in their course.

iii. Many irritants (e.g. tobacco smoke) have been found to potentiate anti-basement membrane antibody deposition in rabbit lungs. In patients with Goodpasture's syndrome, smoking is independently predictive of alveolar haemorrhage.

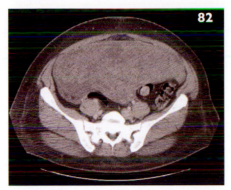

82 A 47-year-old Latina female presented with a 2-week history of shortness of breath. She had recently gained weight. Examination showed dullness at the right lung base, and a full abdomen, which was non-tender. Blood tests were unremarkable, and the chest X-ray showed a very large right pleural effusion. Pleural aspiration showed a protein of 5.2 g/dl, with lactate dehydrogenase of 137 IU/dl and normal cells. Her abdominal CT (**82**) is shown. What is the possible diagnosis?

83 i. How would you manage a young man presenting with this chest radiograph (**83**) for the first time?
ii. What is the risk of recurrence?
iii. How would you manage this?

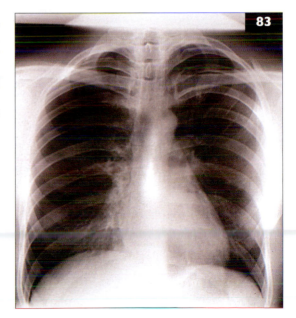

82 A biopsy of a pelvic mass was performed, which showed a lipoleiomyoma with prominent vascularity and degenerative changes. There was focal serositis with mesothelial hyperplasia involving the tumour surface. Focal infarction with sclerosis and oedema was seen, but there was no evidence of malignancy. This is pseudo-Meigs' syndrome.

Meigs' syndrome is the triad of ascites and pleural effusion that develops in association with benign ovarian tumours (most commonly fibromas). The syndrome is called pseudo-Meigs' when the ascites and pleural effusions develop in association with other ovarian or uterine pathology (most commonly malignant tumours). As with Meigs' syndrome, the pleural effusion resolves after removal of the pelvic mass. Benign pathologies included in Meigs' syndrome include fibromas (91%), granulosa cell tumours (5%), and cystadenomas. Pseudo-Meigs' was initially described in a patient with a uterine leiomyoma in 1909. Findings on thoracentesis are consistent with either transudative or exudative effusion. Rarely, the effusion will be haemorrhagic. Diagnosis is made by exploratory laparotomy with sampling of the pelvic pathology.

83 i. The majority of spontaneous pneumothoraces occur as a result of rupture of subpleural apical blebs in otherwise fit and healthy individuals. Rarely there is an underlying inflammatory or degenerative disease process such as TB, scleroderma or interstitial pulmonary fibrosis that requires attention. If the rupture of a small bleb results in a small pneumothorax (<20%) and the patient is asymptomatic, then often nothing needs to be done other than advising the patient to reduce activities. In larger pneumothoraces where the patient is breathless, the pneumothorax should be aspirated via a small cannula attached to a 50 ml syringe via a three-way tap introduced into the second anterior intercostal space. A volume of air up to 2.5 l can be aspirated, but the procedure should be stopped earlier if lung is blocking the needle or no more air is coming out with ease. A chest radiograph taken 1 hr later will show if the procedure has been successful. If the lung has not re-expanded, intercostal tube drainage should be undertaken. Most patients will have their lung re-expanded rapidly and will leave hospital within 5 days. If there is a persistent air leak after this time, surgery should be considered.

ii. The risk of recurrence after a first, conservatively treated pneumothorax is of the order of 30–40%.

iii. A second pneumothorax should lead to consideration of surgery. The operation of choice is a pleurectomy using VATS. VATS may also be used to resect or staple subpleural bullae that may have been responsible for the pneumothorax. Mechanical pleurodesis by pleural abrasion may also be carried out.

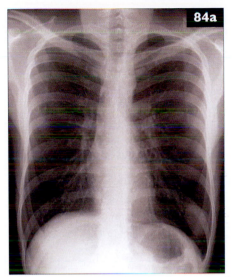

84 A 35-year-old male was referred by his family physician, who noted that he was centrally cyanosed but otherwise well. The following respiratory function test results were obtained:
- Oxygen saturation on air: lying 94%, standing 89%.
- FEV_1 93% expected.
- FVC 97% expected.
- DL_{CO} normal.

The chest X-ray (**84a**) showed a large, well-defined, rounded lesion in the left lower zone. The patient had been treated 10 years previously for a brain abscess.

i. What is the term that describes the oxygen saturation results?
ii. What is the likely diagnosis?
iii. What other problems may occur?
iv. How can the pulmonary lesions be treated?

85 i. What are the main causes of central sleep apnoea?
ii. What are the main symptoms?
iii. How would you treat this condition?

84 i. Orthodeoxia.

ii. PAVM. An upright posture increases the right-to-left shunt through the PAVM and therefore results in a fall in oxygen saturation. A PAVM also allow minor episodes of bacteraemia to reach the arterial circulation and can therefore occasionally lead to brain abscesses. A CT pulmonary angiogram demonstrates a feeding pulmonary artery as the cause of the patient's shunt (**84b**).

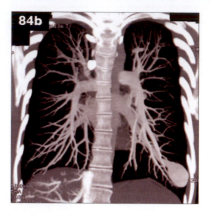

iii. Iron deficiency anaemia due to blood loss from mucosal arteriovenous malformations in the gut.

iv. PAVMs can be effectively treated by embolization of the feeding vessel.

85 i. The most common causes of central sleep apnoea are congestive heart failure and neurological diseases. Central hypoventilation is caused by:
• Primary central hypoventilation.
• Brainstem infarction.
• Encephalitis.
• Arnold–Chiari malformation.
• Chronic opioid treatment.
Causes of neuromuscular respiratory dysfunction include:
• Muscular dystrophy.
• Spinal atrophy.
• Amyotrophic lateral sclerosis.
• Acid maltase deficiency.
Causes of unstable respiratory drive include:
• Sleep onset (transient).
• Hyperventilation-induced hypocapnia.
• Hypoxia (pulmonary disease, high altitude).
• Congestive heart failure.
• Disorders of the CNS.
• Chronic opioid treatment.

ii. Patients may have a diminished sense of breathlessness when hypercapnic. Restless sleep is common, as is daytime somnolence and morning headache. Right-sided heart failure and polycythaemia occur in advanced cases.

iii. Treatment for central apnoea includes supplemental oxygen, nasal CPAP, BiPAP, and respiratory stimulant medications. Nocturnal ventilatory assistance may become necessary by face mask or via a tracheostomy.

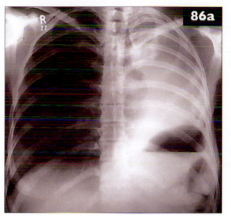 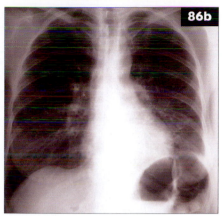

86 These radiographs (**86a, 86b**) are from a patient who has undergone laser resection of a tumour occluding the left main bronchus.
i. What has happened?
ii. What predictive factors are there for this occurring?

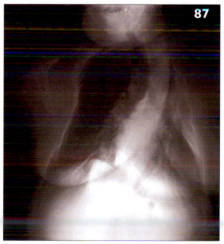

87 **i.** What operation has this patient undergone (**87**)?
ii. Why is there a scoliosis?

86 i. There has been re-expansion of a totally collapsed lung due to removal of the endobronchial part of the tumour. Improved breathlessness and lung function occur, and improved ventilation and perfusion of the previously collapsed lung can be demonstrated by radionuclide scans. It may also permit the drainage of infected retained secretions.

ii. It is difficult to predict which patients will have such an improvement. Where a tumour has progressed radiographically from the periphery towards the hilum, the obstruction is unlikely to respond to a removal of the proximal part of the tumour by laser. A shorter duration of collapse (up to 3 months) is more likely to respond to attempts at re-expansion. During the procedure, it may be difficult to know how far distally an obstruction extends; a CT scan can sometimes help in this regard. An attempt should be made early in the procedure to pass through the obstruction and assess the patency of the distal airways. If these are occluded, the likelihood of a favourable outcome is small.

87 i. Left thoracoplasty. The most common indication for this operation was TB in the pre-chemotherapy area to collapse the lung in the face of progressive or uncontrolled advance of the TB. The patient would initially have been treated by an artificial pneumothorax, often for up to 1 or 2 years – also reducing the aerobic environment that the *Mycobacterium tuberculosis* organism enjoys. It was performed in 1–3 stages developed to discern the extent of patient tolerance of the procedure.

Other methods used to achieve the same result were plombage (plastic spheres inserted extrapleurally inside the chest) and oleothorax (installation of paraffin wax). Thoracoplasty may rarely be performed now in patients who have chronic lung cavities with ongoing systemic symptoms, usually due to infection by resistant organisms, or in patent pleural spaces with failure of the lung to expand and fill the space.

ii. Scoliosis can develop after thoracoplasty in prepubertal patients, and its severity is related to the number of ribs removed. The scoliosis is convex to the side of the surgery. Spinal TB may also have been a concomitant feature in such patients.

Patients with this type of chest wall deformity are at risk of nocturnal hypoventilation, particularly when there is accompanying chronic obstructive airways disease (as many of these patients continue to smoke). Ultimately, hypercapnic respiratory failure (hypoxaemia with hypercapnia) and pulmonary hypertension develop, requiring oxygen at night and non-invasive ventilatory support often just at night.

88 A 51-year-old male with severe COPD had an FEV_1 24% of that predicted, an exercise tolerance of only a few yards on the flat, and a resting PO_2 of 6 kPa. He underwent a procedure to improve his survival and quality of life.
i. Describe his chest X-ray appearances (**88**).
ii. What procedure has he had done?
iii. What are the most common indications for this treatment?

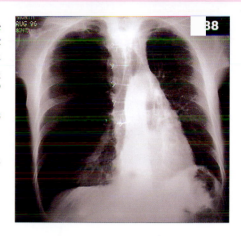

89 A 28-year-old male had chemotherapy for relapsed acute myeloid leukaemia 25 days before presenting with a several day history of coryzal symptoms followed by a dry cough. On examination, he was pyrexial at 37.5°C, and had bilateral widespread inspiratory squeaks and crepitations. His oxygen saturation was 92% on air. This is a representative slice of the CT scan (**89**) performed to identify the cause of the patient's fever, cough, and hypoxia.
i. What does the CT scan show?
ii. What is the likely diagnosis?
iii. What investigations need to be performed?
iv. How should the patient be managed?

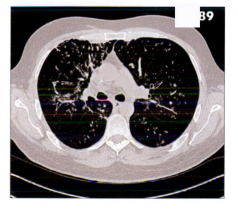

88 i. The chest X-ray shows a marked asymmetry in appearance of the lung fields. The right lung is hyperinflated with a paucity of lung markings. The left lung appears normal. There is also evidence of a previous sternotomy.
ii. The patient has undergone a single (right) lung transplant.
iii. The most common conditions that require lung transplantation are COPD/emphysema (particularly due to α_1-antitrypsin deficiency), cystic fibrosis, bronchiectasis, pulmonary fibrosis, and primary pulmonary hypertension.

Patients must be below the age of 60 and meet stringent criteria. In the case of COPD, the patient's post-bronchodilator FEV_1 must be <25% and the resting PO_2 <7.5 kPa. Hypercapnia and secondary pulmonary hypertension are often present. Many patients have a rapid decline in FEV_1 or life-threatening exacerbations necessitating transplant. In practice, most transplants are for patients with emphysema, cystic fibrosis, or primary pulmonary hypertension, because of their younger age, better resilience, and lesser co-morbidity.

89 i. The CT scan shows 'tree-in-bud' changes suggestive of a small airways inflammatory process, i.e. a bronchiolitis.
ii. These appearances in this context suggest the patient has a respiratory virus infection, which can cause more severe and prolonged disease in an immunocompromised host than in a healthy host. Bronchiolitis is common and can develop into a pneumonia. The viruses seen in this context are respiratory syncytial virus, parainfluenza, influenza, adenovirus, rhinovirus, coronavirus, and the recently identified and characterized respiratory virus metapneumovirus. Similar appearances can occur with *Mycoplasma pneumoniae* and *Chlamydophila pneumoniae* infection, and *Aspergillus* can cause a tracheobronchitis with localized 'tree-in-bud' areas on the CT scan.
iii. Along with routine blood tests, and sputum and blood cultures, tests to identify respiratory viruses are necessary. These can be cultures from nasopharyngeal aspirates or BAL fluid, but a much more rapid diagnosis can be achieved by direct immunofluorescence or PCR of the same samples. This patient had parainfluenza-3 infection confirmed by direct immunofluorescence of a nasopharyngeal aspirate.
iv. Effective antiviral therapies against respiratory viruses are limited. Influenza can be treated with amantidine and the neuraminidase inhibitors zanamivir and oseltamivir, and respiratory syncytial virus with ribavirin or the monoclonal antibody palivizumab, but the efficacy of most treatments is debatable. Treatment is often just supportive with oxygen and antibiotics against associated bacterial infections. The patient needs to be isolated from other immunocompromised patients to avoid patient-to-patient spread.

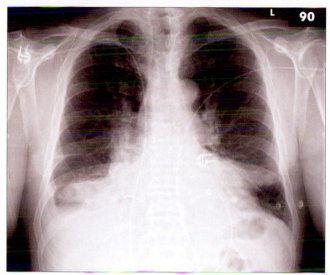

90 A 58-year-old male with a history of asthma had developed progressive fatigue, malaise, dyspnoea, fever, chills, night sweats, and decreased intake over the previous few weeks. He denied cough, chest pain, haemoptysis, orthopnoea, and paroxysmal nocturnal dyspnoea. Two days prior to admission, he had developed a non-pruritic rash on his forearms, buttock, and groin. Current medications included montelukast, rabeprazole, ranitidine, digoxin, betamethasone nasal spray, and tiotropium. On examination, he had bilateral cervical and inguinal lymphadenopathy, and a non-blanching, erythematous macular rash over the groin, buttock, and both forearms. His white cell count showed 23% eosinophils. His chest X-ray is shown in **90**. He underwent a VATS biopsy that showed eosinophilic vasculitis, hyperinflation, and mild, medial hypertrophy of the pulmonary arteries.
i. What is the likely diagnosis?
ii. What are the causes of this?
iii. Describe the treatment and prognosis.

90 i. This is Churg–Strauss syndrome. Churg–Strauss syndrome is an uncommon condition that shares certain clinical and pathological features with Wegener's granulomatosis and polyarteritis nodosa. It is characterized by granulomatous inflammation and a necrotizing eosinophilic vasculitis and necrosis that can affect any organ system but most commonly involves the heart, lungs, skin, nervous system, and kidneys.

ii. The cause of Churg–Strauss syndrome is not known. Its development after allergic hyposensitization, vaccination, exposure to certain drugs, the withdrawal of corticosteroids, and pulmonary infections suggests that these events may initiate the inflammatory cascade. The use of leukotriene antagonists in patients with asthma has been associated with the development of Churg–Strauss syndrome perhaps because it allows for a tapering of corticosteroids and thereby unmasks the syndrome. Other suggested explanations include that it might be an allergic response to the leukotriene antagonist itself or that the use of antagonist produces an imbalance in leukotriene receptor stimulation.

Diagnosis is suggested when a previously healthy patient presents with allergic rhinitis or recurrent sinusitis associated with asthma, followed by signs and symptoms of a systemic vasculitis. The diagnosis is often initially missed as asthma and sinus disease are common in the population. The mean latency between the development of asthma and/or sinusitis and Churg–Strauss syndrome is 8 years.

The 1990 American College of Rheumatology Diagnostic Criteria are:
1. Asthma.
2. Eosinophilia >10% in peripheral blood.
3. Neuropathy, mononeuropathy, or polyneuropathy.
4. Pulmonary infiltrates.
5. Paranasal sinus abnormalities.
6. Extravascular eosinophil infiltration on biopsy.

ANCA positivity is seen in up to 70% of patients, usually with a perinuclear staining pattern. The cytoplasmic pattern has been observed but is rare.

iii. Corticosteroids are the first-line treatment and are usually sufficient for those who do not have severe organ involvement. Cyclophosphamide is generally used when patients relapse or for those with severe necrotizing disease. Plasma exchange, intravenous immunoglobulin, and alpha-interferon have been posited as adjunctive therapies, but no randomized trials inform their use in Churg–Strauss syndrome. Prior to the use of corticosteroids, mortality was approximately 50% within 3 months from vasculitis. The survival rate with corticosteroid therapy approaches 90% at 1 year, 62 to 75% at 5 years, and 50% at 7 years. Factors that define a poor prognosis and increased mortality include renal disease, gastrointestinal involvement, cardiomyopathy, CNS involvement, a weight loss of over 10% body weight, and age over 50 years.

Test	Before treatment	8 hr after treatment
FiO_2	0.4	0.6
pH	7.31	7.29
$PaCO_2$	7.2 kPa	7.9 kPa
PaO_2	8.9 kPa	8.6 kPa
HCO_3	22 mmol/l	21 mmol/l

91 A 70-year-old female with known COPD has been admitted with a fever, purulent sputum, and disorientation.
i. Describe her arterial blood gases before and after 8 hr of nebulized bronchodilators, steroids, and antibiotics (*Table*).
ii. What should be the next step in her management, and what is the physiology behind this intervention?
iii. How successful is it?

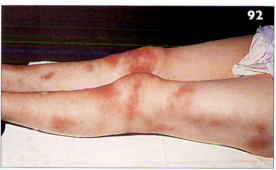

92 This 45-year-old white female presented with bilateral hilar lymphadenopathy on chest radiograph and this painful rash (**92**).
i. What is this syndrome called?
ii. What is her prognosis?
iii. What other cutaneous manifestations may occur in this disease?

91 i. The arterial blood gases demonstrate an acute respiratory acidosis (low pH and raised $PaCO_2$). Despite treatment with bronchodilators, steroids, and antibiotics, she has deteriorated. The PaO_2 has dropped even though the inspired oxygen concentration has been increased.

ii. Non-invasive ventilation should be the treatment of choice. The $PaCO_2$ is inversely proportional to the patient's minute volume (tidal volume x respiratory rate). Non-invasive ventilation improves the patient's minute volume, reducing $PaCO_2$ and therefore improving the pH.

iii. Non-invasive ventilation is successful in approximately 80% of cases but fails in 20%, in particular in those with evidence of pneumonia on chest X-ray. When instituting non-invasive ventilation, it is therefore important to make a clear plan covering what to do in the event of deterioration, and ceilings of therapy should be agreed. The assessment of whether patients with COPD are suitable for elective endotracheal intubation and invasive ventilation is complex and should include functional status, BMI, oxygen requirement when stable, previous admissions to intensive care, age, lung function, and, whenever possible, a careful discussion with other family members.

92 i. Löfgren's syndrome, after a Swedish physician who described it in 1946. It consists of bilateral hilar lymphadenopathy and the rash of erythema nodosum. Lymphoma and granulomatous infections should be considered. An elevated serum ACE may reduce the need for a biopsy confirmation in the absence of atypical features. The syndrome usually occurs in young females who often present with fever, malaise, arthralgias, and painful lesions on their legs (probably due to circulating immune complexes). The condition occasionally relapses and is uncommon in males.

ii. This female is in the best prognostic group of white individuals, with a 90% chance of spontaneous remission of her sarcoidosis within 2 years without corticosteroids. The erythema nodosum should fade within weeks.

iii. Cutaneous involvement with sarcoidosis may occur on the anterior surface of the legs with erythema nodosum. The most common additional skin manifestations are papulonodular lesions. Nodules are smooth reddish-brown and often solitary or in small groups, whereas papules are often numerous and often occur on the face or neck. Lupus pernio occurs mainly in older females and more commonly in black individuals, and is associated with chronic fibrotic sarcoidosis. Although often located across the nose and cheeks, these violaceous plaques may be found on the arms, buttocks, and thighs. Nasal septal perforation may occur. The condition is treated with prednisolone and weekly methotrexate. Sarcoidosis also has a predilection for scars and tattoos and can cause subcutaneous nodules.

93 i. What is this?
ii. When should it be used?
iii. What are the contraindications to its use?

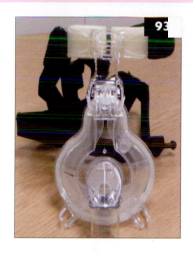

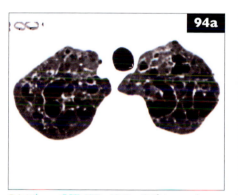

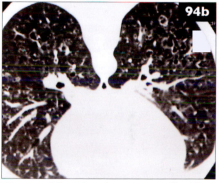

94 These HRCTs (**94a, 94b**) are from a 37-year-old male who presented with a spontaneous pneumothorax.
i. What diagnosis do the HRCTs suggest?
ii. What is the typical clinical presentation of this disease?
iii. What abnormalities are seen on histopathological examination?

93 i. This is a face mask used for non-invasive ventilation. It is tight-fitting, and when attached to a ventilator can provide bi-level (different inspiratory and expiratory) respiratory support. There is a separate port via which oxygen can be entrained.

ii. In the acute setting, it should be considered in patients with hypercapnic respiratory failure and respiratory acidosis due to an exacerbation of COPD. The patient should be conscious and able to co-operate and maintain his or her airway.

iii. An undrained pneumothorax is an absolute contraindication to this treatment. Relative contraindications include copious upper airway secretions, confusion, upper gastrointestinal surgery, bowel obstruction, and haemodynamic instability. BiPAP is commonly employed in patients who are deemed unsuitable for intensive care admission and patients with heart failure or pneumonia in whom standard treatment has failed.

94 i. Eosinophilic granuloma. The major findings on chest CT are irregular, cystic structures of variable size, most being 3–5 cm in diameter (**94a**), suggestive of eosinophilic granuloma. The chest radiograph in this disorder is characterized by diffusely increased interstitial markings. A nodular or reticular nodular infiltrate is present, sometimes accompanied by cystic lesions (**94b**). The infiltrate is most commonly found in the lung periphery and in the upper lobes. Volume loss is characteristically absent on both the chest radiograph and the CT.

ii. Primary pulmonary histiocytosis X or eosinophilic granuloma of the lung can present at any age but is most frequently seen in the third and fourth decades of life. Patients complain of cough and exertional dyspnoea but may be asymptomatic. Spontaneous pneumothorax is a classical association. A progressive decline in lung function and the occurrence of multiple pneumothoraces implies a poor long-term prognosis. Pleurodesis may be of use in these patients. Immunosuppressive treatment is of unproven value. The eosinophilic granulomas can also occur in the pituitary gland, causing diabetes insipidus, and may cause asymptomatic bone cysts, detected on a radiological skeletal survey.

iii. The classical pathological findings are discrete parenchymal nodules composed of fibrous tissue, eosinophils, and 'histiocytosis X' cells, which resemble the Langerhans cells of the skin. The histiocytosis cells are characterized by intracytoplasmic X bodies, which can be visualized by electron microscopy.

95 Shown here is the chest radiograph (**95**) of a 56-year-old female from southeast Asia with chronic cough, malaise, and weight loss. Multiple sputum specimens submitted for mycobacterial and fungal culture have yielded negative results.
i. What are the radiographic findings?
ii. What is the most likely diagnosis, and how can this be established?
iii. What is the appropriate treatment?

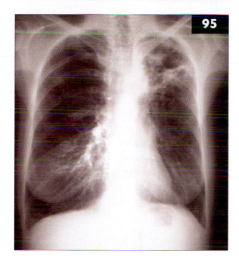

96 A 60-year-old male presents with a mucoid cough that has lasted for 4 months and increasing dyspnoea. He has never smoked. The chest X-ray (**96**) is abnormal.
i. What is the likely diagnosis?
ii. How would you make the diagnosis?
iii. What is the best treatment?

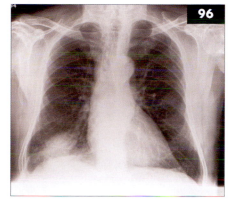

95 i. There is a cavitating infiltrate in the apical segment of the left upper lobe.

ii. Melioidosis is an important cause of respiratory infection in tropical regions, especially south-east Asia. It is caused by the Gram-negative bacterial pathogen *Burkholderia pseudomallei*, acquired by cutaneous inoculation with haematogenous spread to the lungs.

Melioidosis may present acutely, with evidence of cellulitis at the inoculation site, prominent systemic and respiratory symptoms, and diffuse pulmonary infiltrates. A more insidious or chronic form of the disease may develop long after an infected patient has left the endemic area. The presentation of chronic melioidosis is characterized by indolent wasting symptoms, cough, and apical infiltrates that may become fibrotic or cavitating, features indistinguishable from those of pulmonary TB. The diagnosis of melioidosis should be considered whenever a compatible syndrome develops in a patient who has been in an endemic area. The organism can readily be cultured from respiratory secretions or other sites, and infection can be confirmed by serological testing.

iii. *B. pseudomallei* is sensitive to a variety of antimicrobial agents, but resistance is variable and antibiotic selection should be based on *in vitro* sensitivity testing. For acute disease, combination intravenous therapy including an aminoglycoside is recommended for 1 month, followed by several months of oral treatment. For chronic disease, a 3–6-month course of an oral agent such as trimethoprim/sulfamethoxazole (co-trimoxazole) or amoxicillin–clavulanate may be used.

96 i. The chest X-ray shows a reasonably well-defined infiltrate, which lacks density in the right lower lobe. This appearance is compatible with an alveolar cell carcinoma.

ii. Many patients with this tumour produce sputum, often in large quantities. Sputum cytology is therefore often positive. Alternatively, a bronchoscopic transbronchial biopsy will yield the diagnosis.

iii. Alveolar cell carcinomas are a variant of adenocarcinoma, and their histology is often a mixture of these cell types. The tumour can be localized and peripheral, and classically shows air bronchograms. This presentation may be resectable and will in general have a better survival, stage for stage, than an adenocarcinoma. However, if the tumour appears more diffuse on staging CT, it rapidly spreads to the lung lymphatics, to the hilar glands, and to the other lung. At presentation, CT may reveal small areas of contralateral ground-glass shadowing that are likely to be tumour spread. Resection will not be possible. The tumour responds poorly to chemotherapy, despite having a less aggressive nature and, classically, a low standardized uptake value on PET scans.

97 A 65-year-old lorry driver is seen in Accident & Emergency with a 5-hr history of progressive weakness of his arms and legs, along with a dry mouth and some difficulty swallowing. He has a 40 pack–year smoking history and was previously well. Routine blood tests are normal, but the chest X-ray (**97**) is abnormal.

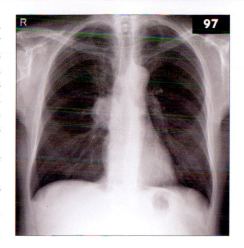

i. What is the likely diagnosis from the chest X-ray?

ii. What are the presenting symptoms due to?

iii. How would you treat this condition?

Test	Result	Reference range
FiO_2	0.6	
pH	7.44	7.35–7.45
PCO_2	4.9 kPa (37 mmHg)	4.6–6.0 kPa (35–46 mmHg)
PO_2	11.1 kPa (83 mmHg)	12 – 16 kPa (91–122 mmHg)
HCO_3	19 mmol/l	22–30 mmol/l

98 A 21-year-old female with a history of asthma presents to the Accident & Emergency department with severe breathlessness.

i. Interpret these arterial blood gas tensions (*Table*).

ii. How should the patient be managed?

97 i. The chest X-ray shows a large centrally placed mass that is in fact situated behind the hilum in the apical segment of the right lower lobe. This is a tumour mass.

ii. The patient has a proximal myopathy with absent tendon reflexes. This, together with the dry mouth and abnormal chest X-ray, makes LEMS likely. This paramalignant syndrome is rare and occurs with small-cell lung cancer; it may precede the clinical or radiological appearance of the tumour by several months. The reflexes can return for some minutes after forced repetitive contracture of the affected muscle groups. An electromyogram will show post-tetanic potentiation.

iii. Treatment is aimed both at the underlying carcinoma, which should be treated by cytotoxic chemotherapy, and at the symptoms of LEMS. The tumour's response to chemotherapy will often, by itself, cause the myopathy to improve. Specific treatment is with high-dose oral prednisolone, 40–60 mg/day, and 2–4 mg/day aminopyridine, which is an anticholinergic antagonist. These drugs can be reduced as a response is seen. The return of LEMS usually heralds the relapse of the primary tumour. It is thought that LEMS carries a better prognosis for survival from the small-cell cancer.

98 i. The patient has a severe exacerbation of asthma causing the PaO_2 to be much lower than expected for an $FiO2$ of 60%. The arterial blood gases show a very wide alveolar–arterial oxygen gradient. This is calculated by applying the alveolar air equation, which gives an assessment of oxygen shunt. The equation is $PaO_2 = FiO_2 - PaCO_2/R$ (where R is assumed to be 0.8). So, here $PaO_2 = 60 - 4.9/0.8$, which $= 60 - 6 = 54$. And therefore PAO_2 (54 kPa) $- PaO_2$ (11.1 kPa) $= 42.9$ kPa.

The normal alveolar–arterial oxygen gradient breathing room air is 2 kPa, and a subject breathing 60% oxygen would have a PaO_2 of approximately 45–50 kPa. Applying a PaO_2 of 45 kPa to the alveolar air equation gives an alveolar–arterial oxygen gradient of 2–3 kPa; i.e. normal gas exchange is occurring. The pCO_2 is within the normal range, which suggests that the exacerbation is severe as one expects a low pCO_2 in patients with acute asthma due to the increased ventilatory drive.

ii. The patient is best managed on a high-dependency unit. Treatment should include high-flow oxygen, continuous nebulized bronchodilators, intravenous hydrocortisone followed by oral prednisolone 60 mg daily, and intravenous magnesium. If the condition does not improve, intravenous aminophylline should be considered. A chest X-ray should be performed to exclude a pneumothorax and pneumonia.

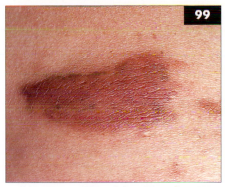

99 i. What is shown in this image (**99**) of the skin of an HIV-positive male?
ii. How may this condition affects the lungs?

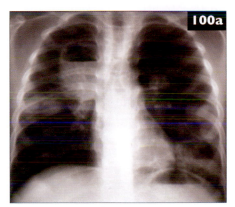
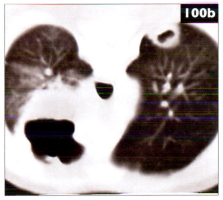

100 Shown are the chest radiograph (**100a**) and CT scan (**100b**) of a 36-year-old man from Romania whose has been complaining of back pain and a cough for 6 weeks, but is otherwise well.
i. What are the radiographic abnormalities?
ii. What is the most likely diagnosis?
iii. How can this diagnosis be established?

99 i. The photo shows discrete, raised red-purple patches resulting from Kaposi's sarcoma. AIDS-related Kaposi's sarcoma occurs principally in homosexual or bisexual men infected with the recently identified human herpes virus-8. Unlike classical forms of the disease, AIDS-associated Kaposi's sarcoma frequently involves lymph nodes, gastrointestinal tract, and lung, commonly in the setting of extensive cutaneous disease and very rarely as an isolated event. Kaposi's sarcoma typically occurs in advanced HIV disease when the CD4-positive count is below 100 cells/µl.
ii. Pulmonary Kaposi's sarcoma may cause radiographic infiltrates and respiratory symptoms that mimic a variety of other infectious and neoplastic processes. Dyspnoea and cough are the most common presenting symptoms. Fever and night sweats may be present and commonly suggest a concomitant infection. Haemoptysis may also occur and heralds a poor prognosis. Evidence of parenchymal infiltrates on a CT scan in the presence of visceral Kaposi's sarcoma may be sufficient for the diagnosis. The lesions of Kaposi's sarcoma may also be readily identified endobronchially. However, biopsy is not recommended due to a high risk of haemorrhage. In selected cases, open lung biopsy may be necessary.

100 i. There are large spherical lesions with smooth margins in both lungs. CT scanning confirms that these are thin-walled, fluid-filled cysts.
ii. Cystic abnormalities of this size are most likely the result of hydatid infection. Pulmonary sequestrations may occasionally manifest in this fashion, as may infected bullae or bronchogenic cysts. Sequestrations are almost always in the lower lobes.
iii. Hydatid disease results from the ingestion of eggs of the ubiquitous carnivore tapeworms *Echinococcus granulosa* or *E. multilocularis*, prevalent in areas where dogs coexist with the natural intermediate hosts (i.e. sheep and cattle). Oncospheres released in the gut enter the portal circulation, and larvae then develop in the liver, lungs or, less commonly, other systemic sites. *E. granulosa* larvae form encapsulated cysts (cystic hydatid disease) that grow slowly and cause symptoms only if they rupture, become secondarily infected, or reach sufficient size to compress adjacent structures. The chest radiograph typically shows one or more homogenous masses with sharply defined margins. The 'lily pad' sign may be present if air enters the cyst. This results from collapsed cyst walls and debris floating on the surface of the fluid. Eosinophilia may be present, but serological tests are not always positive unless a cyst has ruptured. CT, and particularly MRI scanning, can reveal the cystic nature of these lesions and can identify coexistent hepatic cysts. Needle biopsy of suspected hydatid cysts should be *avoided*, and treatment by intact surgical excision is desirable because a spillage of cyst contents can cause anaphylaxis and may lead to larval dissemination. *E. multilocularis* cysts fail to mature, and the invading scolices cause continued inflammation and tissue destruction (alveolar hydatid disease). Pulmonary involvement is focal or diffuse and treatment with systemic antihelminthic drugs (e.g. praziquantel or mebendazole) is recommended.

101 i. Describe the different types of exercise apparatus used for progressive exercise testing.
ii. What is a progressive exercise test, and why is it done?

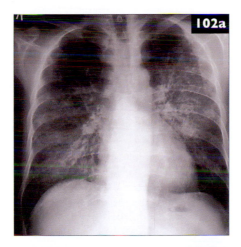

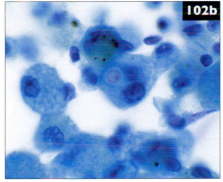

102 Fever, cough, and dyspnoea were the presenting features of this male patient's illness (**102a**). His CD4-positive lymphocyte count is 0.08x10^9/l.
i. Describe the cytological finding in the BAL specimen (**102b**), and give the diagnosis of his condition.
ii. What is a more common presentation of disease caused by this agent?
iii. Discuss the management of this condition and any potential complications.

101 i. The different types of apparatus used for progressive exercise tests are a stepping test, or more commonly a treadmill test, and a cycle ergometer test. During these tests, the workload is increased by small increments at regular time intervals. The workload will gradually increase until the patient reaches his or her maximum exercise capacity or maximal oxygen uptake.

ii. The main purpose of a progressive exercise test is to measure the work capacity achievable by the individual. Several measurements can be made, including heart rate, minute ventilation, and mixed expired gas concentration by capturing the expired gases with the patient breathing through a two-way valve box via a mouth piece. It is mandatory to measure the ECG during exercise and, from it, the heart rate. Minute ventilation can be measured by collecting expired gas volumes or by sampling the expired gas volumes for the expired carbon dioxide and oxygen concentration; from this, the oxygen uptake per unit time (usually minute by minute) is measured.

The progressive exercise test is commonly used in the investigation of heart disease (e.g. the Bruce protocol), looking for chest pain, ECG abnormalities, and breathlessness. In patients with lung disease, exercise is usually stopped by maximum exercise ventilation being achieved, causing breathlessness. It is also possible to measure arterial blood gases during exercise, either by an indwelling arterial cannula or from arterialized capillary blood collected from an earlobe. Measurements of arterial/arterialized blood gas tensions will allow the alveolar arterial oxygen gradient to be calculated.

102 i. This encapsulated intracellular yeast is typical of *Cryptococcus neoformans*. This can be confirmed by antigen testing of the blood and the culture of blood and BAL fluid. Other yeasts that cause lung disease include *Candida* sp. and *Histoplasma capsulatum*, but these can be distinguished on morphology and culture.

ii. A subacute meningitis would be the most common presentation of illness caused by this organism in AIDS.

iii. Cryptococcal infection is treated with intravenous amphotericin B, sometimes with the addition of flucytosine in more severe cases. Alternatively, fluconazole (orally or intravenously) is used for less severe cases. High-dose treatment is given for 4–6 weeks, followed by long-term secondary prophylaxis – usually with oral fluconazole. The response to treatment response in usually monitored by clinical parameters and falling cryptococcal antigen titres. Respiratory disease may lead to respiratory failure, and meningitis can progress to widespread involvement of the brain (cryptococcomas) and hydrocephalus.

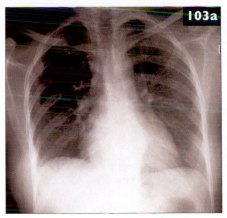

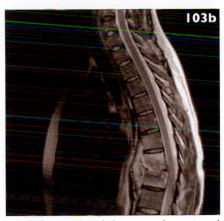

103 A 25-year-old Eritrean female presented with a 6-month history of continual back pain, but no other symptoms. These are her chest radiograph and the MRI of her spine.
i. What are the abnormalities present on the chest radiograph and on the spinal MRI?
ii. What is the likely diagnosis?
iii. How should the patient be managed?

104 This male patient has a tender lump in his chest wall (104) that has appeared over the past 2 weeks. He had a VATS pleurodesis for a malignant pleural effusion 2 months ago.
i. What is the likely diagnosis of the underlying malignancy, and what is the lesion?
ii. How would this now be treated, and could it have been prevented?

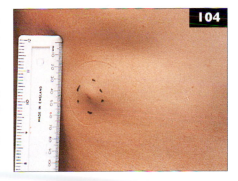

103 i. The chest radiograph shows a left paravertebral mass parallel to the thoracic vertebrae behind the heart. The MRI scan shows destruction of the T8/T9 disc space, the presence of a large prevertebral abscess and a posterior extradural mass and oedema of the T8 and T9 vertebral bodies. There is also a distinct angulation of the spine at this point but no overt cord compression.
ii. This is Pott's disease, i.e. TB of the spine. The patient comes from a high-risk population, and the combination of disc involvement, spinal angulation, and an associated soft tissue mass are very suggestive of TB infection.
iii. The patient needs a biopsy/aspiration of the soft tissue mass to prove the diagnosis and obtain material for microscopy and culture for *Mycobacterium tuberculosis* to help confirm the diagnosis and allow antibiotic sensitivity testing. She should be started on standard antituberculous therapy, and neurosurgical advice should be sought to ensure her spine is stable and to minimize the risk of cord compression. As tuberculous masses can swell when treatment is initiated and the tuberculous lesions are very close to her spinal cord, there is a case for combining antituberculous treatment with oral corticosteroids (e.g. prednisolone 60 mg once daily initially, which is roughly equivalent to 30 mg due to the effects of rifampicin [rifampin] on the metabolism of corticosteroids) to prevent neurological deterioration on starting treatment.

104 i. The lesion is a skin metastasis from either an adenocarcinoma of the lung or a mesothelioma. Both these diseases commonly present with breathlessness due to a large pleural effusion. This is best treated with pleurodesis and, at the same time, biopsy under VATS. Pleurodesis is effective in preventing a recurrence of the effusion in 80% of cases. An alternative would be a medical (or intercostal drainage and instillation of talc) pleurodesis after an initial pleural aspiration has revealed malignant cells. However, medical pleurodesis is successful in only 50% of individuals.
ii. The treatment of the skin nodule will be by one or two fractions of radiotherapy. Skin metastases are a frequent complication of penetration of the chest wall in the presence of a malignant pleural condition. These lesions can be painful and may not be adequately controlled by radiotherapy. It is now routine practice to administer radiotherapy prophylactically to any drain, needle, or VATS scar as soon as possible, which prevents this complication.

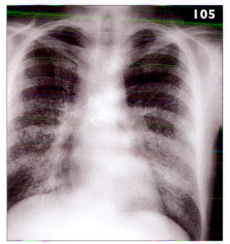

105 This is the chest radiograph (**105**) of a 39-year-old male who is known to be HIV positive. He has presented with fever, headache, and a dry cough. The patient was born in Arizona but moved to the Pacific North-West at age 27 years.
i. What does the chest X-ray show?
ii. What is the significance of the geographical history?
iii. How would you investigate this patient to exclude the diseases associated with his geographical history?

106 A 28-year-old male with asthma is brought to Accident & Emergency by ambulance. He has the following features:
• An inability to complete sentences.
• Pulse 120 beats/min.
• PEFR 40% of that predicted.
• Respiratory rate 28 breaths/min.
What additional features would be present in a life-threatening attack?

105 i. The chest X-ray shows widespread military nodular shadowing in both lungs, with hilar lymphadenopathy.

ii. The appearances on the chest radiograph would suggest TB, but with this geographical history endemic fungal pathogens could also cause this presentation. In particular, for people who have lived in the south-west of the USA or northern Mexico, infection with *Coccidioides immitis* should be considered.

The inhalation of fungal spores is usually asymptomatic but can cause a (usually) self-limiting illness termed 'valley fever' with fever, cough, arthralgia, and a rash. However, even the asymptomatic inhalation of spores can result in latent infection for many years, which can, if the patient becomes immunosuppressed, e.g. HIV infection, develop into active disease. This can then disseminate, with widespread infection affecting the lungs, joints, skin, and CNS. Treatment requires systemic antifungal therapy with amphotericin B or itraconazole.

Similar diseases occur with *Histoplasma capsulatum* (associated with central USA, Mexico, Puerto Rica, and parts of South Asia), *Paracoccidioides braziliensis* (South and Central America), and *Blastomyces dermatitidis* (central North America, Mexico, Middle East, Africa, and South Asia).

iii. Latent infection with endemic mycoses can be diagnosed by serological testing. Infection requires the identification of fungal spores in sputum, CSF, joint effusions, or histopathology specimens by microscopy (silver or PAS staining) or prolonged culture.

106 These features alone suggest a severe exacerbation of asthma. The clinical features of a life-threatening attack are shown in the *Box*.

If an attack is not adequately relieved, the patient can become exhausted and be unable to sustain adequate minute ventilation. The silent chest may be due to exhaustion, causing inadequate pleural pressure generation to inspire. Lack of wheeze therefore may be a sinister and not a reassuring sign. Cyanosis, especially when receiving high-flow oxygen, is potentially catastrophic. Bradycardia and confusion can also indicate incipient collapse.

Features of a life-threatening asthma attack
- Silent chest
- Cyanosis
- Bradycardia
- Exhaustion, confusion
- Respiratory acidosis
- PEFR <33% predicted

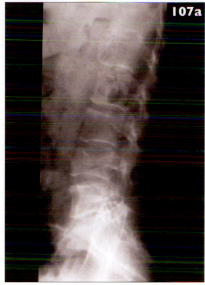

107 A patient with known carcinoma of the bronchus presents with a 2-day history of progressive mid-lumbar back pain and numbness on the anterior surface of his left thigh. Shown here (**107a**) is a lateral radiograph of his lumbar spine.
i. What is the likely cause of the symptoms?
ii. How would you investigate them?
iii. How would you treat this patient?

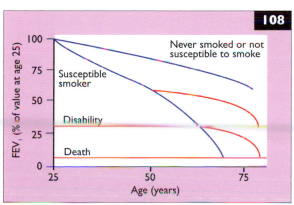

108 i. What does this plot (**108**) show?
ii. How does this affect the patient's outcome?

107 i. The back pain is mostly likely to be due to metastatic disease. The vertebral column is one of the most common sites of metastatic spread.

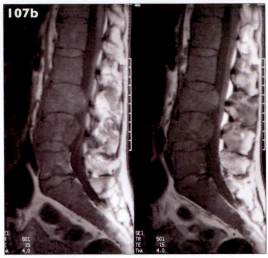

ii. The numbness of the thigh may indicate a root lesion (lower motor neurone) compatible with early corda equina compression. Enquiries into bladder and other sphincter function is essential. The patient needs plain radiographs of the lower thoracic and lumbar spine. Even if these are normal, further investigation is needed, and this should be by urgent MRI scan to visualize the cord and surrounding bony structures. Tumour is best identified by MRI, as would be a soft tissue mass of other cause, e.g. TB (**107b**).

iii. Suspected paraparesis needs urgent treatment. Paraplegia, once established, rarely improves. The primary treatment is radiotherapy together with steroid cover. There is no advantage from surgical decompression. In patients with small-cell lung cancer for whom a cord lesion is the presenting symptom, chemotherapy can be added following radiotherapy if the clinical response appears adequate.

108 i. This plot shows the rates of decline of FEV_1 in healthy individuals and in smokers.

ii. FEV_1 is a strong predictor of survival in COPD. The normal rate of decline is about 27 ml/year, i.e. 1,000 ml in 40 years. The rate is generally accelerated in smokers, up to a maximum of 140 ml/year. The plot shows how the rates of decline allow disability to manifest at younger ages, depending on both the rate of decline and individual habitual activity. Whereas a healthy person will never develop pulmonary disability, the heavy, susceptible smoker will become affected in his 50s or 60s. Note that quitting may result in the rate of decline reverting to that of a never-smoker, delaying or preventing the onset of disabling symptoms. The plot shows premature death due to loss of lung function at a considerably earlier age than normal.

It is also likely that an impaired growth of lung function in childhood and adolescence as a result of recurrent infections or passive exposure to tobacco smoke may lead to lowered maximally attained lung function in adulthood, such that the individual starts to decline from a lower threshold than normal.

109 A 57-year-old male has persisting exertional dyspnoea and hypoxia 4 weeks after discharge from intensive care. He had been admitted to the intensive care department with a severe right upper lobe pneumonia that was complicated by ARDS and required ventilation for 22 days. These are his lung function test results.

Lung function results:
FEV_1	2.14 (70% expected)
FVC	2.59 (67% expected)
DL_{CO}	38% expected
K_{CO}	64% expected

i. What could be causing this patient's persisting dyspnoea?
ii. What investigations are necessary?
iii. What is the natural history of this problem?

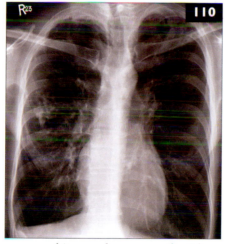

110 A 44-year-old, non-smoking male presented with several weeks' cough, dyspnoea, and purulent sputum on the background of longstanding asthma. He was apyrexial and not systemically unwell. **110** is the chest X-ray on presentation. His FEV_1 was 1.9 l/s (expected 4.2 l/s) and his FVC 3.6 l (expected 5.4 l). No acid-fast bacilli were seen on microscopy of multiple sputum samples, all of which were negative for acid-fast bacilli and remained negative for mycobacteria after 8 weeks of culture of culture. A full blood count and blood chemistry were normal except for a total IgE level of 7143 kIU/ml.

i. What does the X-ray show, and what possible diagnoses need to be considered?
ii. How should the patient be investigated?
iii. What is the treatment of the most likely diagnosis?

109 i. The lung function tests show a restrictive spirometric defect and a markedly reduced transfer factor, which would be compatible with post-ARDS lung fibrosis. Another cause of dyspnoea, usually after more prolonged ventilation, is a tracheal stenosis caused by intubation and tracheostomy, but this would cause an obstructive defect and a characteristic flattened appearance to the inspiratory part of the flow–volume loop.

ii. As well as lung function tests and a chest X-ray, an HRCT scan is necessary and should show the characteristic subpleural changes of interstitial fibrosis. In contrast to the distribution of the airspace shadowing in early ARDS, which is gravity dependent and therefore often most marked posteriorly in patients ventilated supine, post-ARDS fibrosis is often more marked anteriorly.

iii. In up to 70% of those who survive an episode of ARDS, lung function returns to within the normal range.

110 i. The chest X-ray shows hyperinflated lungs, ring shadowing with associated patchy shadowing in the right middle zone, and a streaky infiltrate in the left upper zone.

ii. Opacities in the upper zones can be due to primary lung cancer, TB, and non-tuberculous mycobacterial infections, lung abscesses, unusual infections such as *Nocardia*, actinomycosis, endemic fungi, melioidosis and *Aspergillus*, and inflammatory conditions such as vasculitis or necrotizing granuloma. However, the combination of poorly controlled asthma, massively elevated total IgE levels, ring shadows suggestive of bronchiectasis, and pulmonary opacities indicate that allergic bronchopulmonary aspergillosis is the likely diagnosis.

Investigations should be directed to identifying allergic bronchopulmonary aspergillosis and excluding the other causes. Patients with allergic bronchopulmonary aspergillosis can have a moderate eosinophilia ($>1000/mm^3$), almost always have positive skin prick tests to *Aspergillus* and a markedly raised IgE level (>1000 IU/ml), and usually have positive *Aspergillus*-specific IgE in their serum (although less often positive *Aspergillus* precipitins, e.g. IgG). *Aspergillus* can be identified by culture or cytology in sputum or bronchial washings, and the patient may expectorate characteristic plugs of sputum shaped like casts of the bronchi. A CT scan can, in advanced cases, demonstrate bronchiectasis, usually proximal, and mucous plugging of the large and small airways (the latter giving a 'tree-in-bud' appearance).

iii. The treatment of allergic bronchopulmonary aspergillosis requires treatment of the asthma and airways obstruction component using high-dose inhaled and often oral corticosteroids, as well as bronchodilators. In addition, infective exacerbations of the bronchiectasis require treatment with 10–14 days of appropriate antibiotics. Prolonged treatment with the antifungal agent itraconazole 200 mg twice a day can reduce the dose of oral prednisolone for patients on long-term corticosteroids. Itraconazole is poorly absorbed, especially in patients with achlorhydria, and drug levels should be monitored.

111 i. What is the impact of OSA on mortality?
ii. What is thought to be the risk factor associated with these nocturnal deaths?

112 i. What percentage of the dose is inhaled into the lungs from an MDI?
ii. What are the advantages of using a large-volume spacer?

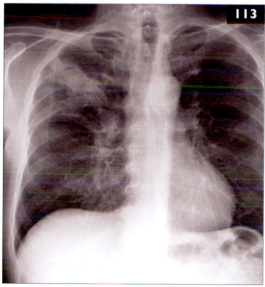

113 This chest X-ray (**113**) is from a 65-year-old male with right shoulder pain and malodorous breath. The condition improved following 6 months of oral penicillin. What is the likely diagnosis?

111 i. OSA raises the mean 24-hr blood pressure by at least 4–6 mmHg in those with an apnoea–hypopnoea index of >20/hr. OSA has been demonstrated in several studies to be associated with a 20% greater risk of myocardial infarction and a 40% increase in stroke. However, the effect of OSA on mortality has not been well measured. One study has demonstrated that conservatively treated patients, compared with those treated by tracheostomy, had nearly a five times the risk of cardiovascular- or stroke-related death. The effects of OSA on mortality are not clear. In diabetes, increased apnoeas and hypopnoeas are associated with an increase in insulin resistance independent of obesity.

ii. The lack of autonomic nervous system control during rapid eye movement sleep may represent a risk period for health and may be a precipitating factor in nocturnal death.

112 i. The average dose entering the lungs from a well co-ordinated inspired breath with the MDI is about 10%. The rest are either large particles that impact on the throat, or particles less than 5 µm size that do not deposit in the lung airways or alveoli and are exhaled. Deposition patterns using depot DPIs are similar. The ideal particle size for optimal lung deposition is around 5 µm.

ii. The advantages of using a spacer is that patient co ordination with the firing of the MDI becomes less important. Also, as the drug leaves the MDI at 97 km/hr (60 mph), timing the inhalation is more important than when the chamber is used to 'collect' the actuation. There is better deposition in the lung from a spacer, rising to 12–14%, and with more going to the lung periphery than with the MDI alone. Fewer large particles leave the chamber, and oral thrush rates are far less.

113 This is thoracic actinomycosis. It is a subacute-to-chronic bacterial infection caused by filamentous, Gram-positive, anaerobic bacteria that are not acid fast. It is characterized by the formation of multiple abscesses and sinus tracts that may discharge sulphur granules and commonly invade the pleura and chest wall. The condition arises following the aspiration of oropharyngeal secretions that contain actinomycetes. The chest X-ray shows dense consolidation in the right upper lobe with volume loss. It mimics the appearance of lung cancer but may be cured with a prolonged course of penicillin of at least 6 months.

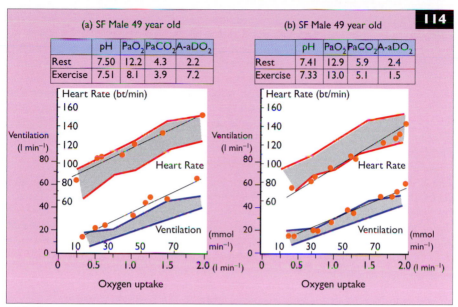

114 Shown (**114**) is the response of heart rate and ventilation to increasing oxygen uptake during a progressive work rate test in a male with alveolar proteinosis. Exercise has stopped with the heart rate at the upper limit of normal and a ventilation that was higher than normal but not at predicted maximum, and the patient was complaining of breathlessness. The subsequent exercise test followed a procedure that improved the patient's breathlessness.
i. Comment on the two exercise test results.
ii. What was the procedure that improved the patient?

115 i. What are the symptoms of OSA?
ii. What is the Epworth Sleepiness Score, and how predictive of the severity of OSA is it?

114 i. 114a shows excessively high ventilation from the beginning of exercise to the completion of the test. Arterial blood gases show hypoxaemia with increasing hypoxia at the end of exercise and a widened alveolar arterial oxygen gradient (A–aDO$_2$, from 2.2 to 7.2 kPa). The post-treatment exercise test (**114b**) shows a considerable improvement in resting heart rate and the heart rate response during exercise, and the ventilatory response remained within the normal range. The arterial PO_2 and the alveolar arterial oxygen gradients were considerably improved. **ii.** The procedure that improved the patient was a BAL of 10 l, which is the treatment of choice in flushing out the abnormal protein from the alveolar spaces in these patients.

115 i. The main symptoms of OSA are: excessive daytime sleepiness, difficulty concentrating, daytime fatigue, unrefreshing sleep, nocturia, depression, nocturnal choking, and decreased libido. They occur especially in overweight, middle-aged males who have often snored for years. OSA is also related to collar size, and increasing neck circumference with weight gain is more common in males because females who gain weight tend to accumulate it around their hips. **ii.** The Epworth Sleepiness Score (*Box*) is a useful guide to detecting OSA but is in itself insufficient. Partners will often score the patient differently, and the highest score should then be recorded. Many sleepy patients do not score very highly. However, there is a good relationship between greater scores on the Epworth Sleepiness Score and CPAP compliance. A score greater than 12 is very suggestive of OSA.

Epworth Sleepiness Score: How often are you likely to doze off or fall asleep in the following situations, in contrast to feeling just tired? This refers to your usual way of life in recent times. Even if you have not done some of these things recently, try to work out how they would have affected you. Use the following scale to choose the most appropriate number for each situation:

0. Would never doze
1. Slight chance of dozing
2. Moderate chance of dozing
3. High chance of dozing

- Sitting and reading
- Watching TV
- Sitting, inactive in a public place (e.g. a theatre or a meeting)
- As a passenger in a car for an hour without a break
- Lying down to rest in the afternoon when circumstances permit
- Sitting and talking to someone
- Sitting quietly after lunch without alcohol
- In a car, while stopped for a few minutes in traffic   Total   /24

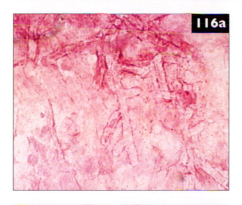

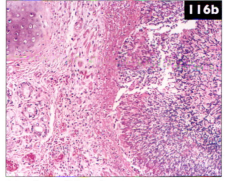

116 i. What do these histology slides show?
ii. Who gets this disease?
iii. What is the treatment?

117 A 74-year-old male with a clinically operable carcinoma is being considered for surgery. What are the minimally acceptable lung function parameters for a lobectomy and for a pneumonectomy? Consider spirometry, gas transfer, and exercise testing in your answer.

116 i. The dichotomous branching hyphae of an *Aspergillus* species invading lung tissue – the diagnosis is invasive aspergillosis. The morphology of the fungus helps to identify the species as an *Aspergillus*, but precise identification requires culture. The most common *Aspergillus* species causing lung infection is *A. fumigatus*, which is responsible for about 70% of infections. Other *Aspergillus* species that cause lung disease include *A. flavus*, *A. terreus*, and *A. niger*. Less common moulds that have a presentation similar to that of invasive aspergillosis include *Fusarium*, *Scedosporium*, and *Penicillium*.

ii. Invasive aspergillosis is largely a disease affecting those who are immunosuppressed, especially those who have prolonged and profound neutropenia. It is therefore especially common in patients with haematological malignancies or aplastic anaemia, and in bone marrow transplant recipients. It is also common in lung transplant patients and occurs in other organ transplant patients as well as patients with AIDS with very low CD4-positive cell counts. A less aggressive indolent form can affect patients with pre-existing lung disease and lesser degrees of immunosuppression such as those with diabetes or patients on corticosteroids.

iii. Treatment is with systemic antifungal agents such as amphotericin, caspofungin, and voriconazole. Although effective, amphotericin frequently has to be discontinued due to toxicity (especially renal) and has been largely superseded by liposomal formulations, which are much better tolerated. The introduction of caspofungin and the newer azoles such as voriconazole has improved treatment options for invasive fungal infections enormously. However, recovery from invasive aspergillosis is highly dependent on the patient's immune status improving, and mortality is up to 50%.

117

- Because males and females of similar ages have different lung capacities, and because these are also affected by height and weight, all predictions of postoperative lung function from preoperative values should be expressed and considered as a percentage of that predicted.
- If the preoperative FEV_1 and DL_{CO} are both >80% predicted, a pneumonectomy is possible. If either is <80%, an exercise test measuring VO_2max is necessary. If the VO_2max is <10 ml/kg/l and the FEV_1 or DL_{CO} is <40% predicted, a lobectomy will not be possible.
- If the VO_2max is >20 ml/kg/l or the FEV_1 or DL_{CO} is >75% predicted, a pneumonectomy will still be safe.
- However, for those with intermediate results, i.e. FEV_1 or DL_{CO} 40–75% of that predicted and VO_2max 10–20 ml/kg/l, split lung function tests are needed, e.g. a *V/Q* scan. This will determine the distribution of blood and air to the lung tissue planned for resection. If the lung tissue remaining after resection would contain <40% of function, no resection is possible. Above 40% a lobectomy is possible.

118 i. What is this condition (**118**)? How can the arms and legs be affected, and how is the condition seen here recognized?
ii. What else is it associated with?

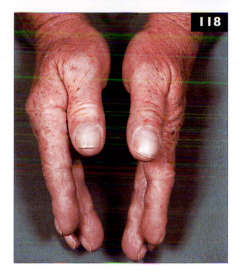

119 Describe the changes in late pregnancy that occur in lung volumes, ventilation, and respiratory muscle pressures.

120 This 50-year-old female developed a fever and dyspnoea with oxygen saturations of 88% on air 3 days after an abdominal operation. **120** shows her chest X-ray.
i. What is the likely diagnosis?
ii. What investigations are necessary?
iii. How should the patient be managed?

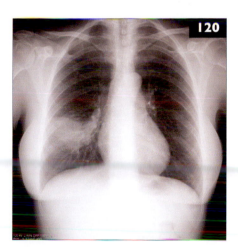

118 i. The hands show clubbing with a loss of the nailfold angles. This is associated with non-small-cell lung cancers. It can be associated with pain and swelling of the distal forearm and shins, which can become red and oedematous, and the bones themselves very tender to pressure. Radiography will show new bone formation or periostitis. The condition is known as HPOA. Bone scintigraphy with Tc-99m-methylene diphosphonate may reveal increased tracer uptake along the distal fingers and toes owing to clubbing. Treatment is with non-steroidal anti-inflammatory medication, with, if possible, treatment of the primary tumour.

ii. HPOA occurs primarily with lung cancer but has also been reported in association with pulmonary sepsis, thymic carcinoma, chronic myeloid leukaemia, thyroid carcinoma, Hodgkin's disease, adenocarcinoma of the oesophagus, primary lymphocarcinoma of the lung, and bronchial carcinoid tumour. Benign associations include cyanotic congenital heart disease, pleural fibroma, Graves' disease, oesophageal achalasia, portal cirrhosis, inflammatory bowel disease, leioma of the oesophagus, cystic fibrosis, and idiopathic or familial HPOA.

119 In late pregnancy, the diaphragm is pushed cephalad by up to 4 cm. The potential loss of lung capacity is partially offset by increased anteroposterior and transverse diameters. However FRC and RV are reduced, and TLC may fall a little. Diaphragmatic and maximal mouth pressures remain normal.

Minute ventilation increases markedly from the first trimester and reaches 20–40% above baseline at term. This is mainly due to an increase in tidal volume. A respiratory alkalosis with compensated renal excretion of bicarbonate results, with $PaCO_2$ falling (3.8–4.3 kPa). The PaO_2 remains normal.

120 i. Hospital-acquired pneumonia with or without atelectasis (areas of subsegmental pulmonary collapse).

ii. A full blood count, arterial blood gases, blood and sputum cultures, and blood biochemistry are necessary.

iii. The patient should be given oxygen, kept well hydrated, and encouraged to sit up rather than lie in bed to help respiration and minimize basal atelectasis, which will impair gas exchange. Physiotherapy may help the patient to clear tenacious sputum. She will need empirical antibiotics to cover the usual organisms that cause hospital-acquired pneumonia, which are initially *Streptococcus pneumoniae*, *Staphylococcus aureus*, and Gram-negative coliforms. However, in patients who have been in hospital for a long period or in intensive care, the spectrum of causative organisms extends to include antibiotic-resistant coliforms and *Pseudomonas aeruginosa*.

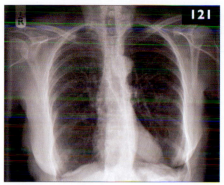

121 This 40-year-old smoker is complaining of increasing exertional dyspnoea.
i. What does the chest X-ray (**121**) suggest?
ii. Is this condition hereditary, and if so, how?
iii. What is the mechanism of the developing pathology?
iv. What advice can you offer the patient? What are the family implications?

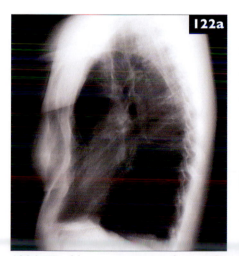

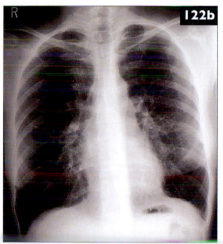

122 i. Would you expect any abnormality of the VC of this 18-year-old male patient whose lateral (**122a**) and posteroanterior (**112b**) chest X-rays are shown?
ii. What associated clinical abnormalities might this patient have?

121 i. The chest X-ray shows larger than normal lung fields with darker than normal bases, cystic bi-basal shadowing, and vascular pruning in both lower lobes, suggestive of basal emphysema.

ii. This condition α_1-antitrypsin deficiency emphysema is an autosomally recessive inherited disease. It occurs in 1 in 5,000 children in the UK and 1 in 2,700 in the USA. More than 75 biochemical variants of α_1-antitrypsin have been described. They have given rise to the Pi inhibitor nomenclature. The most common allele is PiM, and the most common genotype is PiMM, which occurs in 86% of the normal UK population. PiMZ and PiS are the next two most common genotypes and are associated with α_1-antitrypsin levels of 15% and 75% of normal PiMM levels. The threshold point for developing emphysema is 35–50% of normal level. The homogygous PiZZ type shows levels that are 10–20% of the average normal value, and this is the strongest genetic risk factor for panacinar emphysema.

iii. α_1-Antitrypsin is a major inhibitor of serine proteases, including neutrophil elastase, and has its greatest affinity for the enzyme neutrophil elastase. It is synthesized in the liver, and in cases of deficiency, it remains entrapped in the liver as PAS-staining granules. A deficiency of the enzyme leads to unrestrained proteolytic damage to the lungs, leading to emphysema, which develops at an earlier age than the common variety seen in COPD. The damage occurs at the lung bases as this is where blood flow and air (plus tobacco irritants) mix maximally. Cigarette smoking is a co-factor for α_1-antitrypsin deficiency emphysema, probably as a result of oxidation and hence inactivation of the remaining functional α_1-antitrypsin by oxidants of cigarette smoke.

iv. The most important advice is to stop smoking. The family should be screened by measuring α_1-antitrypsin serum levels, and homogyzotes and heterozygotes should be identified and advised never to smoke. Heterozygotes usually do not get the disease even if they do smoke, but advice should be given about having children if the partner is also a heterozygote.

122 i. The lateral chest X-ray shows pectus excavatum, an inward displacement of the sternum that has probably been present from birth. Despite being what is occasionally a striking physical abnormality, it does not cause reduction of the VC except in a minority of cases. In addition, such patients do not have breathlessness due to the sternal deformity.

ii. Associated features include thoracic kyphosis and scoliosis. Cardiac effects include right axis deviation on ECG (due to leftward displacement of the heart), supraventricular tachycardias, mitral valve prolapse, and, rarely, reduction of right ventricular filling due to cardiac compression.

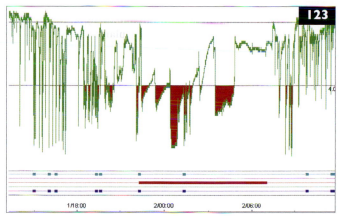

123 A 50-year-old male has a 9-month history of a dry cough. He is otherwise well. Lung function and chest radiology are within normal limits.
i. What is this investigation (**123**)?
ii. What does it show?
iii. List the common causes of chronic cough

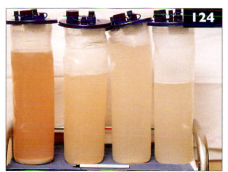

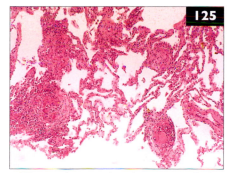

124 i. The material in **124** was obtained from whole-lung lavage of a patient with what disorder?
ii. What is the appropriate treatment for this condition?
iii. Do corticosteroids have a therapeutic role?

125 i. What is the diagnosis of this transbronchial biopsy (**125**), and what is the differential diagnosis?
ii. Why is this condition easy to diagnose by transbronchial biopsy?
iii. Which other conditions may be confidently diagnosed by transbronchial biopsy?

123 i. The investigation is ambulatory oesophageal pH monitoring, which is the most sensitive and specific investigation for the diagnosis of gastro-oesophageal reflux.

ii. The test demonstrates low pH in the oesophagus consistent with gastro-oesophageal reflux disease, which is an important cause of chronic cough and occurs in up to 40% of individuals with a cough lasting more than 3 months.

iii. The *Box* shows the common causes of chronic cough.

> **Causes of chronic cough with a normal chest X-ray**
> - Gastro-oesophageal reflux
> - Oesophageal dysmotility
> - Asthma syndromes
> - COPD
> - Rhinitis
> - Drugs, e.g. ACE inhibitors

124 i. The lavage fluid shown is characteristic of pulmonary alveolar proteinosis, a disorder in which a phospholipid-rich proteinaceous material is deposited in the alveoli and bronchioles without associated lung fibrosis. Lung fluid obtained from whole-lung lavage or BAL is milky in appearance and contains large macrophages with prominent cytoplasm.

ii. Whole-lung lavage is the only treatment that is consistently successful. Lavages of as much as 20 l total fluid washed in are often performed at one session under general anaesthesia. The procedure is generally well tolerated and may be repeated as necessary, generally at 6–12-month intervals.

iii. Corticosteroids have not been shown to have a beneficial effect in this disorder and may be harmful. Inflammation does not appear to play a role in the pathogenesis. The condition is often self-limiting, with spontaneous remission on radiography after lavage clearance.

125 i. The compact granulomas with a paucity of interstitial inflammation are typical of sarcoidosis.

ii. The granulomas are situated adjacent to the bronchi, making them amenable to diagnosis by bronchial or transbronchial biopsy. Only four separate biopsies are usually needed to obtain typical granulomas. A transbronchial lung biopsy may be positive even when the chest radiograph shows only hilar lymphadenopathy without parenchymal shadowing. The main differential diagnosis is EAA, although in that condition the granulomas are not as tightly formed and are overshadowed by an interstitial inflammatory cell infiltrate.

iii. Other conditions that can be readily diagnosed with transbronchial lung biopsy include lymphangitis carcinomatosa and alveolar proteinosis. Conditions such as idiopathic pulmonary fibrosis may be suggested by transbronchial biopsy, but the definitive diagnosis usually requires large samples such as from an open lung biopsy.

126 i. Would the management of asthma in a pregnant patient differ from usual asthma treatment?
ii. How would pregnancy be affected by asthma?
iii. What is the effect of pregnancy on asthma?

127 A 75-year-old female with a 50 pack–year smoking history has a 2-month history of cough, sputum production, and fevers.
i. Describe the findings on her CT (**127**).
ii. What is the likely diagnosis, and how would you confirm it?
iii. What is the treatment?

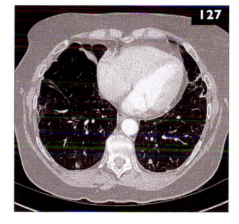

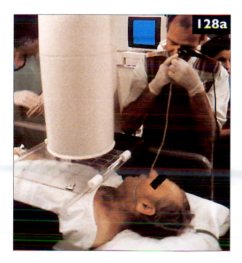

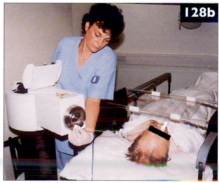

128 i. What procedure (**128a, 128b**) is this patient undergoing?
ii. What side-effects may result from this treatment?

126 i. No, although there should be increased vigilance over asthma control, especially close to the time of delivery. Delivery is usually uncomplicated if control is good. As with all asthmatics, inhaled therapy is preferred. No increased teratogenesis has been reported when mothers receive beta-agonists, inhaled steroids, sodium cromoglicate (cromolyn), or theophylline. When systemic steroids are used, neonatal hypoadrenalism is very rare.

ii. A prospective study of 504 pregnant asthmatic women showed that, of 177 patients not initially treated with inhaled corticosteroids, 17% had an acute attack, in contrast to 4% of the 257 patients who had been on inhaled anti-inflammatory treatment from the start of the pregnancy. No differences were observed between the two groups in terms of length of gestation, length of the third stage of labour, or amount of haemorrhage after delivery. Nor were any differences observed between these groups with regard to relative birthweight, incidence of malformations, hypoglycaemia, or need for phototherapy for jaundice in the neonatal period. In an earlier smaller prospective study of 198 pregnant women, there was a small increase in pre-eclampsia and a higher incidence of caesarean section in asthmatic patients compared with those without asthma.

iii. There is no specific effect. In about 40–50% of females, asthma remains unchanged, in 25% it improves, and in another 25% it deteriorates.

127 i. The CT image demonstrates multiple small nodules on a background of emphysema.

ii. The appearances are typical of non-tuberculous mycobacteria. Pulmonary metastases, vasculitis, and septic emboli are other possible causes. Non-tuberculous mycobacteria, in particular *Mycobacterium avium* complex, may be confirmed from BAL. *Mycobacterium avium* complex is an uncommon but important cause of morbidity in patients with COPD. DNA probe testing on lavage samples may establish the diagnosis rapidly and exclude TB.

iii. Treatment is with clarithromycin, rifampicin (rifampin), and ethambutol with consideration of additional intravenous amikacin in severe cases. Treatment should continue until the patient has been culture negative on therapy for 1 year. The mortality can be as high as 50% despite good compliance with therapy.

128 i. Endobronchial brachytherapy. Its role is primarily palliative for breathlessness but also for cough and haemoptysis. It is indicated for an endobronchial tumour with a mural and/or endobronchial component, preferably without extrinsic compression. Occasionally, it may be used with curative intent in patients with small endobronchial tumours.

ii. The procedure is performed under local anaesthetic with intravenous sedation and is generally well tolerated.

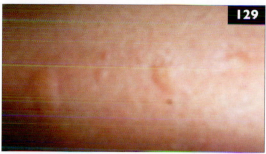

129 i. What does **129** show?
ii. What is the pathological process behind this reaction?
iii. What are the common stimuli that cause it?

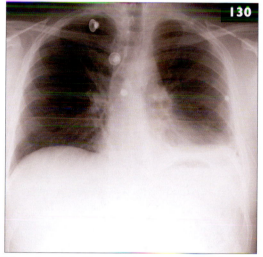

130 A 26-year-old male of Indian origin presents with a 2-month history of exertional breathlessness, fevers, and night sweats.
i. Describe the chest X-ray (**130**) findings.
ii. What investigations would you carry out, and what results would you expect?

129 i. The picture shows a typical wheal and flare reaction.

ii. This is a type 1 (immediate) hypersensitivity reaction. It results from the IgE-mediated release of histamine and other inflammatory cytokines from mast cells and basophils. This process in the skin results in urticaria, characterized by hives or wheals that cause significant pruritis. Angio-oedema is localized tissue swelling that may occur in tissues throughout the body. If it occurs in the upper airway, e.g. larynx or tongue, it can cause life-threatening airway obstruction. IgE-mediated cytokine release in the airways results in asthma, and if the mast cell and basophil products are released systemically, anaphylactic shock can occur.

iii. The most common allergens are peanuts, bee stings, latex, pollen, animal dander, and drugs, e.g. penicillin. Once the causative agent has been identified, meticulous allergen avoidance is the most important intervention. Anaphylactoid reactions are clinically similar to anaphylaxis and are due to mast cell degranulation but are not IgE mediated. Common examples include the reactions to radiocontrast dyes and opiates.

130 i. The chest X-ray shows a left-sided pleural effusion with increased density at the left hilum. The most likely diagnosis is TB.

ii. Pleural aspiration will reveal a lymphocytic exudate with a low glucose level. Samples should be sent for culture for *Mycobacterium tuberculosis*. However, the yield from PCR and culture from tuberculous pleural effusions is relatively low, at 40%. Higher diagnostic yields of over 90% may be obtained with blind pleural biopsy using an Abram's needle. In cases where malignancy is more likely, ultrasound-guided pleural biopsy is the investigation of choice if cytological examination of pleural fluid does not provide the diagnosis. The causes of a lymphocytic pleural effusion are given in the *Box*.

A tuberculous pleural effusion is most commonly caused by a delayed hypersensitivity reaction to the presence of mycobacterial antigens, which responds to antituberculous therapy usually within a few weeks. This should be distinguished from a tuberculous empyema in which pus with a high mycobacterial load occupies the pleural space; this usually requires percutaneous drainage.

Causes of a lymphocytic pleural effusion

Malignancy
- Primary lung cancer
- Mesothelioma
- Pleural metastases
- Lymphoma (rare)

Infection
- TB
- Amyloidosis (rare)
- Sarcoidosis (rare)

131 As well as dyspnoea, this male patient also complains that he has had multiple floating spots across his field of vision for several weeks, and on examination he has retinal haemorrhages and exudates (**131a**).
i. How commonly would such eye and pulmonary problems be connected?
ii. What is the appropriate management of this situation?

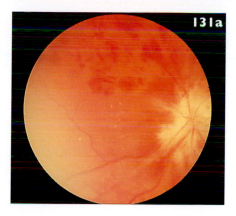

132 A 70-year-old male who is known to have a squamous cell carcinoma of the lung is admitted with a 2-day history of confusion, abdominal pains, vomiting, and constipation.
i. What is the differential diagnosis for his confusion?
ii. What is the likely metabolic cause, and how would you treat it?

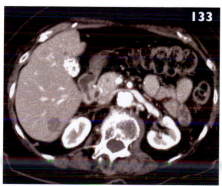

133 i. What does the CT scan (**133**) show?
ii. What is the differential diagnosis?

131 i. The retinal problem (**131a**) is due to CMV. The differential diagnosis of interstitial pneumonitis is as in the answer to **173**, with *Pneumocystis jirovecii* pneumonia (formerly *Pneumocystis carinii* pneumonia, or PCP) still being the most likely cause (**131b**). Other than the eye, this organism also causes disease of the gut, nervous system, and biliary tree. Rarely, CMV may be implicated in HIV-related pneumonitis when other

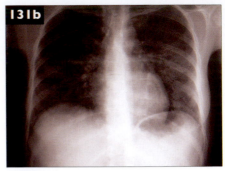

pathogens, such as *P. jirovecii*, have been excluded as a cause.

ii. The initial management would be as in **13**, that is, therapy for presumed *P. jirovecii* pneumonia until the result of bronchoscopy has been obtained. In the rare case of CMV pneumonitis, the patient will be treated with intravenous ganciclovir at high dose for 2–3 weeks. If the CMV pneumonitis occurs without concomitant eye involvement, no further therapy is necessary.

132 i. The common causes of confusion in a patient with known lung cancer are cerebral metastases, poor attention to pain control leading to opiate excess, uraemia, pneumonia, and hypercalcaemia. This patient has a squamous cell carcinoma in which hypercalcaemia can present as a paramalignant syndrome due to the secretion of a cyclic AMP stimulating factor. He does not appear to complain of bony pains, making the hypercalcaemia unlikely to be due to increased bone turnover from multiple metastases.

ii. Hypercalcaemia presents with thirst, polyuria, dehydration, confusion, constipation, and eventually coma. Treatment is by intravenous rehydration, intravenous hydrocortisone, and intravenous bisphosphonate. The latter can be very effective and needs repeating every 4–6 weeks. Treatment of the primary tumour whenever possible is also likely to be beneficial.

133 i. The CT scan shows two darker areas within the liver that are of differing size and likely to be metastases.

ii. The differential diagnosis can often be between malignancy and benign cysts, which are usually smooth in outline and non-contrast-enhancing. An ultrasound scan will discover whether they are fluid-filled cysts or malignant deposits. Liver metastases are usually asymptomatic in newly diagnosed cases of lung cancer, and are found in about 5% of cases of non-small-cell lung cancer thought to be operable. Their presence is more common late in the course of the disease, with up to 60% of autopsy cases having liver deposits.

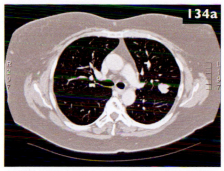
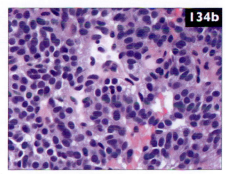

134 A 62-year-old female with a 100 pack–year history had a chest X-ray taken to evaluate her complaint of a chronic, non-productive cough. Pulse oximetry showed an oxygen saturation of 85% when breathing air. Spirometry showed moderate airflow limitation. A left upper lobe nodule was found, leading to a chest CT (**134a**). BAL was negative, and a transbronchial lung biopsy was obtained (**134b**).
i. What does the histology show?
ii. What is the diagnosis?
iii. What is the appropriate treatment?

135 A 55-year-old female presents with a 6-week history of a non-productive cough, fevers, malaise, and some weight loss. There is no improvement with a course of amoxicillin and clarithro-mycin. Her HRCT scan is shown (**135**). A bronchoscopy is normal and shows no evidence of an obstructing lesion, TB, eosinophilia, or bronchoalveolar cell carcinoma.

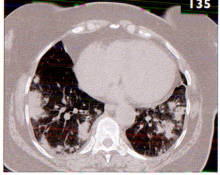

i. Describe the HRCT appearances.
ii. There is clinical and radiological improvement with oral steroids. What is the diagnosis, how may it be confirmed, and what are the possible causes?

134 i. Neuroendocrine tumors can show a variety of histological abnormalities including diffuse hyperplasia, neuroepithelial bodies, carcinoid tumourlets, and typical carcinoid tumour, any or all of which can be associated with airway wall thickening and fibrosis. Neuroendocrine cells are confirmed by their staining with bombesin or chromogranin.

ii. Finding diffuse small nodules (i.e. 2 mm, seen in the right upper lobe on the slice) indicates diffuse involvement, which, in addition to the large carcinoid tumor in the left upper lobe, indicates diffuse idiopathic pulmonary neuroendocrine cell hyperplasia with carcinoid. Diffuse idiopathic pulmonary neuroendocrine cell hyperplasia is felt to be a preneoplastic condition, and the most common physiological deficit observed with it is airway obstruction; several investigators have reported an association with BO.

iii. Treatment is difficult. Cytotoxic agents are ineffective. Octreotide has been tried as it binds to carcinoid tumour cells and inhibits growth as well as the release of hormones. Agents targeting the epidermal growth factor receptor transduction pathway have also been tried since neuroendocrine cells overexpress epidermal growth factor receptors.

135 i. The HRCT shows patchy alveolar opacities that are bilateral and peripheral.

ii. The diagnosis is organizing pneumonia. Inflammatory indices are often raised, but no specific blood tests exist. BAL shows a mixed pattern with increased neutrophils and lymphocytes. The diagnosis may be confirmed by transbronchial or lung biopsy that shows intra-alveolar buds of granulation tissue. The causes of organizing pneumonia are listed in the *Box* and must be excluded. Cryptogenic organizing pneumonia for which no cause is found responds well to oral corticosteroids, usually within 48 hours. The dose may be tapered after 4–6 weeks, but the condition often relapses. Prolonged treatment of 6–12 months is usually required.

Causes of organizing pneumonia

Infection
- Bacteria, e.g. mycobacteria
- Viruses, e.g. influenza
- Parasites, e.g. *Plasmodium vivax*
- Fungi, e.g. *Pneumocystis jirovecii*

Drugs, e.g. amiodarone, methotrexate, phenytoin

Connective tissue disorders, e.g. rheumatoid arthritis, Sjögren's syndrome

Wegener's granulomatosis

Post bone-marrow transplant

Previous exposure of the lungs to radiotherapy (e.g. for breast cancer)

136 A 60-year-old male is admitted with confusion and an abnormal chest X-ray. His electrolytes show a sodium of 119 mmol/l, potassium of 3.7 mmol/l, urea of 2.2 mmol/l, an and osmolality of 255 mOsm/kg.
i. What is happening here, and what is the differential diagnosis?
ii. How do you treat the condition?

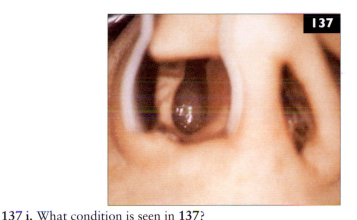

137 i. What condition is seen in **137**?
ii. How is it treated?
iii. What is the common association of this when it occurs in patients with asthma?

136 i. The blood results suggest the syndrome of syndrome of inappropriate ADH secretion. If the chest X-ray shows a mass, a small-cell lung cancer is the most common association of this syndrome with malignancy. The ectopic secretion of ADH causes waterlogging, confusion, and haemodilution of electrolytes with a low serum osmolality (<275 mOsm/kg), together with a concentrated urine and osmolality >200 mOsm/kg. This syndrome is present with abnormal electrolytes in 10% of new presentations of small-cell lung cancer, and 50% will not excrete a waterload. Other causes of this syndrome include pulmonary infections, CNS disorders, and some drugs.

ii. The treatment will include treatment of the primary tumour with chemotherapy and oral demeclocycline, which competes for ADH binding sites in the kidney. Renal function should be monitored and the demeclocycline reduced or stopped once the tumour is responding to therapy.

137 i. A nasal polyp, a red mass in the region of the middle turbinate. These occur when oedematous sinus mucosa prolapses into the nasal cavity. They are often associated with perennial rhinitis and low-grade sinusitis.

ii. Nasal polyposis should be treated medically with a short course of oral steroids or local steroid drops followed by topical steroid sprays. If this is not successful, intranasal or endoscopic polypectomy can be considered for polyps that occlude the nasal cavity. Surgery is not curative, however, and the recurrence rate is greater than 40%. For polyposis that occurs in the setting of chronic rhinosinusitis, the allergic disease should be treated with antihistamines, topical nasal corticosteroids, and immunotherapy.

iii. Some 20–40% of patients with asthma have nasal polyps, and many of these patients are allergic to aspirin (acetylsalicylic acid); 10% of all chronic asthmatics respond to aspirin or other non-steroidal anti-inflammatory drugs with an exacerbation of asthma and acute rhinoconjunctivitis. Some 30% of asthmatics with polypoid rhinosinusitis have aspirin sensitivity. Other allergic causes include fungal infestations, sinusitis and Churg–Strauss syndrome. There can also be infective causes, as well as underlying cystic fibrosis or immune deficiency states. Malignancy is rare.

138 A 29-year-old male was in a motor vehicle accident in which he fractured his femur, right humerus, and liver. No abdominal surgery was needed. On day three of his hospitalization, he developed haemoptysis. His chest CT is shown in **138**. What is the diagnosis?

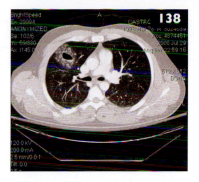

139 A 60-year-old male with a 20 pack–year smoking history has a small haemoptysis on 3 consecutive days.
i. What are the common causes of this, and how often is a diagnosis made?
ii. What tests should be carried out?

140 A 60-year-old male who has never smoked has a longstanding history of a dry cough. Over the last few months, he has become increasingly breathless on exertion.
i. Describe the appearances on the chest X-ray (**140**).
ii. What is the most likely cause of these appearances?
iii. What complications may occur?

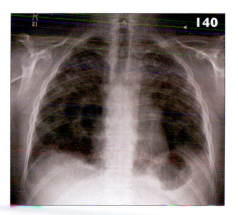

138 Post-traumatic pseudocyst. Blunt chest trauma can result in tears of the lung parenchyma termed post-traumatic pseudocysts or pneumatoceles (pseudocyst being the preferred term since these are epithelium-lined cavities). Post-traumatic pseudocysts are, not surprisingly, more common in young males (average age 17–30 years, with the male:female incidence ratio being as high as 11:1). The most common symptoms are chest pain, dyspnoea, and haemoptysis. Treatment is conservative unless substantial bleeding occurs, in which case wedge resection may be needed. The pseudocysts generally resolve in 1–4 months, larger cysts taking longer.

139 i. In published series, the causes of haemoptysis are neoplasm (12–24% of cases), bronchiectasis (1–40%), bronchitis (7–40%), pneumonia (3–16%), TB (3–6%), unknown (3–22%), and miscellaneous causes (11–26%).
ii. In a male of this age and smoking history, a carcinoma must be excluded. Assuming that the chest X-ray is normal, he should proceed to a CT of the thorax and a bronchoscopy. A chest X-ray may be abnormal in up to 40% of individuals with this type of history. Most neoplasms seen at bronchoscopy will be noted on CT scan, but CT scanning may identify up to 20% of tumours not visible on bronchoscopy because they are peripheral.

140 i. The chest X-ray shows evidence of mid and upper zone fibrosis. The hila are pulled up. The process may also result in lung cavities in the mid-zones.
ii. The most common cause of upper zone fibrosis is sarcoid. However, pneumoconiosis, hypersensitivity pneumonitis, previous TB, histoplasmosis, and seronegative arthropathies must be excluded. Sarcoidosis may be staged by the radiographic appearances (*Box*).
iii. Any lung cavities may be complicated by the development of an aspergilloma. Aspergillomas predispose to life-threatening haemorrhage. The incidence of lung cancer is also increased in the context of pulmonary fibrosis.

Radiographic staging of sarcoidosis
Stage 0: Normal chest radiograph
Stage I: Hilar and mediastinal lymph node enlargement
Stage II: Lymphadenopathy and parenchymal disease
Stage III: Parenchymal disease only
Stage IV: Pulmonary fibrosis

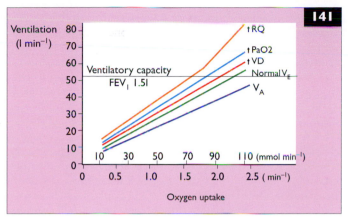

141 i. How is the maximum exercise ventilation predicted in patients with chronic airflow obstruction?
ii. Ventilation for a given oxygen uptake is often excessive in patients with airflow obstruction. What factors contribute to an excessively high ventilation during exercise in these patients and others with pulmonary disease?

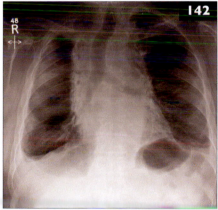

142 A 69-year-old female who has been treated with chemotherapy and mediastinal radiotherapy for non-Hodgkin's lymphoma presents with a 4-month history of dry cough and dyspnoea. On examination, she is apyrexial and has no respiratory signs. She is known to have longstanding pleural thickening of unknown origin. **142** is her chest X ray.
i. What new changes does the chest X-ray show?
ii. What is the likely diagnosis, and how can this be confirmed?
iii. What is the management and outlook?

141 i. The maximum exercise ventilation is predicted as the $FEV_1 \times 35$ in litres.
ii. The ventilatory response to exercise is linear until anaerobic metabolism stimulates ventilation further by a decrease in the pH.

Minute ventilation is a combination of alveolar ventilation and dead space ventilation. In patients with airflow obstruction, the contribution from the dead space, both anatomical and physiological, increases. The worse the airflow obstruction, the higher the minute ventilation has to be in order to maintain a normal alveolar ventilation and rate of gas exchange.

Other factors that will increase minute ventilation are:
- Hypoxia: which will add to ventilatory drive, and ventilation will rise.
- Respiratory exchange ratio: if the patient makes an anaerobic contribution to exercise, either due to an abnormal diet, e.g. high fat or low carbohydrate, or because the anaerobic mechanisms 'kick in' early due to poor aerobic metabolism.

141 shows an idealized scheme where minute ventilation (V_E) comprises alveolar ventilation (V_A), dead space ventilation (VD), and contributions due to hypoxia (PaO_2) and an increase in respiratory exchange ratio (respiratory quotient, RQ). The horizontal line shows the predicted maximum exercise ventilation for an FEV_1 of 1.5 l, and it can be seen that as the various factors cause the minute ventilation to rise, the curves will move to the left, prematurely limiting exercise.

142 i. The chest X-ray shows dense bilateral shadowing adjacent to the mediastinum with sparing of the rest of the lungs. The shadowing has a linear edge.
ii. These appearances are characteristic of post-radiotherapy fibrosis in patients who have been treated with radiotherapy for mediastinal malignancy (e.g. lymphomatous involvement of the mediastinal nodes). The radiological abnormalities have a straight border parallel to the mediastinum with almost complete sparing of the more distal lung. A CT scan will clarify the distribution of the changes and will show ground-glass infiltration with nodules in the early phase, evolving to fibrotic changes with traction bronchiectasis. Radiotherapy pneumonitis usually develops within 3 months of the radiotherapy but can occur much later and is also often exacerbated by subsequent cycles of chemotherapy (so called 'recall' pneumonitis). The patient may have characteristic areas of pigmentation and telangiectasia of the skin overlying the affected area.
iii. Patients with radiotherapy-induced pneumonitis are treated with oral corticosteroids, which may decrease the risk and severity of significant permanent fibrotic damage. However, patients are often left with residual dyspnoea and can in severe cases die from progressive respiratory failure. Disease progress or improvement is best monitored by lung function testing, which will show restrictive lung function impairment with a reduced transfer factor.

143 A 69-year-old male, previously a pipe-fitter, presents with a 4-month history of exertional breathlessness and a dry cough. On examination, he has evidence of digital clubbing and fine inspiratory crackles at both bases.
i. What is the diagnosis?
ii. What aspects in the history and what investigations would confirm your diagnosis?
iii. What management options are available?

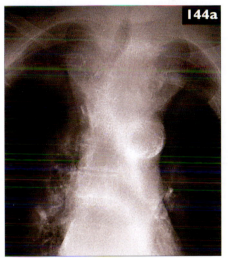

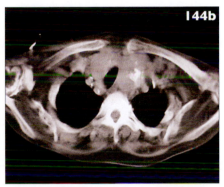

144 An elderly female complained of shortness of breath on exertion but was otherwise in good health.
i. What abnormalities are evident on the chest radiograph (**144a**) and CT film (**144b**), and what is the likely diagnosis?
ii. What further diagnostic tests are likely to be of value?
iii. What risks are associated with this condition?
iv. What management is advisable, and what specific risks should be mentioned to the patient?

143 i. The most likely diagnosis is asbestosis.
ii. In the history, previous exposure to asbestos should be confirmed. Connective tissue disorders should also be excluded, and a detailed drug history should be taken. Pulmonary function tests will show a restrictive defect and reduced transfer factor. An HRCT would show reticulonodular infiltrates at the lung bases. The presence of calcified pleural plaques on the diaphragmatic surface make the diagnosis most likely to be asbestosis. Autoantibody tests will be negative. The diagnosis of asbestosis is usually made clinically, in the absence of other causes of fibrosis, and lung biopsy is not generally required.
iii. Corticosteroids and other immunosuppressants are ineffective, and no other treatments are beneficial. Patients should be advised to stop smoking in view of the markedly increased risk of lung cancer in this situation. Infections should be treated promptly. Patients with a diagnosis of asbestosis should also be informed that they may qualify for financial compensation.

144 i. There is an upper mediastinal mass that is exhibiting areas of calcification (poorly seen on the radiograph). The trachea is markedly deviated. The features are those of a retrosternal thyroid goitre.
ii. None. Radio-iodine scanning is frequently performed but is almost never of value as the goitre will not take up the iodine. Bronchoscopy is non-contributory. Needle biopsy might reveal a thyroid carcinoma, but this would be unlikely to exhibit calcification, and a negative core would not exclude this diagnosis.
iii. Any airway obstruction can worsen with deteriorating exercise tolerance. Haemorrhage can occur into the gland, causing acute enlargement and an airway emergency. Malignant degeneration has very rarely been reported.
iv. Subtotal thyroidectomy is indicated to relieve airway compression. This is usually possible through a collar incision. The chief hazards are damage to the recurrent laryngeal nerves and transient postoperative hypocalcaemia from parathyroid injury. Very occasionally, tracheomalacia may exist, which results in instability of the tracheal wall postoperatively and difficulty with respiration.

145 A 55-year-old, non-smoking female presented with a 6-week history of progressive exertional dyspnoea associated with a dry cough. Nine months previously, she had undergone haematopoietic stem cell transplant for chronic lymphocytic leukaemia, receiving a graft from an unrelated donor. The post-transplant period was complicated by graft-versus-host disease affecting her oropharynx and skin. She was apyrexial. Chest radiographs and CT scans of the lungs were unremarkable. Spirometry showed an FEV_1 of 1.0 l/min and an FVC of 2.0 l. Her transfer factor was normal when adjusted for lung volumes. Prior to the stem cell transplant, her FEV_1 had been close to the expected values for her age and height, at 2.3 l/min and 3.0 l, respectively.
i. What is the likely diagnosis?
ii. How should the patient be managed?

	Predicted	Actual
PEFR (l/min)	590	490
FEV_1 (l)	4.41	3.10
FVC (l)	5.20	4.20
DL_{CO} (mmol/min/kPa)	12.01	11.50
K_{CO} (mmol/min/kPa/l)	1.72	1.69

146 The pulmonary function tests (*Table*) were obtained on a 23-year-old, 225 kg male before a laparoscopic gastrojejunal bypass planned for obesity.
i. What is the pulmonary function test abnormality?
ii. Does the patient have an intrapulmonary cause for a restrictive pulmonary disease (e.g. pulmonary fibrosis)?
iii. What pathophysiological processes contribute to the restrictive pattern seen?
iv. Will these tests improve with weight loss?

145 i. The spirometry values show a marked obstructive defect that had occurred since her allograft bone marrow transplant, a situation that is highly suggestive of BO. BO is a progressive small airways obstructive disorder sometimes associated with bronchiectasis that occurs in 5–10% of bone marrow allograft patients, especially those with graft-versus-host disease affecting other parts of the body. It is thought to be caused by graft-versus-host disease affecting the respiratory epithelium.

ii. The diagnosis is usually clinical as definitive confirmation would require VATS lung biopsy. CT scans of the lungs can be normal or show changes suggestive of small airways disease, with a mosaic pattern, especially on expiratory films. CT evidence of mild bronchiectasis is not uncommon. Active viral infections should be excluded using a nasopharyngeal aspirate or BAL. Treatment is with increased immunosuppression including inhaled steroids, as well as bronchodilators, although the disease is often poorly reversible and can progress to respiratory failure and death. A clinically identical disease is seen in up to 50% of lung transplant recipients, and is a common cause of late death in patients who survive the initial transplant period.

146 i. A restrictive pattern of disease.

ii. These tests are consistent with obesity, i.e. an extrathoracic cause. They would also be compatible with other forms of chest wall disease, such as scoliosis, muscular weakness, or paralysis of the diaphragm. Without further clinical information, no other diagnosis, including that of pulmonary fibrosis, need be sought. For obesity to cause a reduced TLC, the ratio between the weight (in kg) and the height (in cm) must generally exceed 1.0. Reductions in FRC, VC, and RV can occur with lesser degrees of obesity. The gas transfer (DL_{CO}) is normal, but it can also be reduced in the presence of gross reduction of lung volume, although it will correct to normal when alveolar volume is incorporated (K_{CO}). This implies normal pulmonary gas exchange, and a low DL_{CO} is probably due to basal hypoventilation as a direct consequence of the obesity.

iii. Obese individuals have increased chest wall mass, resulting in a reduction in net outward elastic recoil pressure. The compliance of the lung and chest wall falls as weight increases. The increased mass of the abdominal wall and abdominal contents reduces the FRC. Accordingly, these patients develop airway closure in dependent lung zones that becomes most pronounced when the patient lies supine. The changes in PaO_2 observed when these patients lie supine can be great.

iv. Pulmonary function tests improve toward normal as weight is lost.

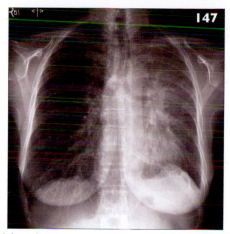

147 This 56-year-old female presents with a week's history of hoarseness and some mild breathlessness. She is otherwise well.
i. What does the chest X-ray (**147**) show?
ii. What is the likely diagnosis, and how would you make it?
iii. What is the significance of the lesion regarding stage of disease?

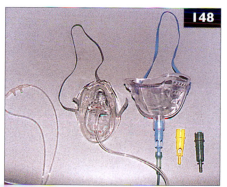

148 What are the indications for use of each of these three oxygen delivery devices (**148**) in the acute setting?

147 i. The chest X-ray shows collapse and consolidation of the left upper lobe characterized by loss of the cardiac outline and increasing opacification and density towards the apex of the lung. There also is evidence of lymphangitis in the right lower lobe, shown as septal lines reaching the periphery.

ii. The likely diagnosis is a lung cancer with the primary in the upper lobe and metastatic spread to the nodes in the left hilum and subaortic fossa, where the left recurrent nerve loops under the aortic arch and is destroyed in that region by tumour. Bronchoscopy will confirm that the left vocal cord is paralysed and often partially adducted, contributing to breathlessness by causing some obstruction to airflow in the trachea. If the primary tumour is seen in the left upper lode orifice, it can be biopsied. If not, a CT scan may show nodes accessible by EBUS-guided transbronchial node biopsy.

iii. Approximately 3–5% of lung cancers can present with hoarseness, and this signifies mediastinal involvement either by direct invasion of the recurrent laryngeal nerve by the primary tumour, or, more commonly, by metastatic nodal involvement. In both circumstances, the tumour will be inoperable, with mediastinal spread of the cancer.

148 Nasal prongs are useful at flow rates of 2–3 l/min for mild hypoxaemia (SaO_2 88–90%). These allow the patient to eat or drink, and there is no carbon dioxide rebreathing. Higher flow rates can be achieved, although this may cause discomfort and dry the nasal mucosa. In addition, the inspiration of oxygen delivered is variable and uncontrolled and therefore potentially harmful.

A Hudson or MC face mask. These can deliver oxygen at flow rates up to 15 l/min, corresponding to an approximate FiO_2 of 0.7. The amount of delivered oxygen is dependent on the rate and depth of the patient's respiration, and the mask is not safe in patients with a reduced hypoxic drive who require controlled oxygen therapy.

A Venturi mask. This enables controlled oxygen (24%, 28%, or 35%) to be delivered at high flow rates. Entrainment of air occurs through the holes in the coloured fittings at the neck of the mask to give the high total flow rate, which may be needed in severely dyspnoeic patients. It is indicated for hypoxaemic patients with a reduced hypoxic drive whose oxygen delivery must be constant to prevent uncontrolled respiratory depression with subsequent hypercapnia. A range of fittings is available, giving a range of inspired oxygen concentrations. Each fitting requires a different oxygen flow rate from the wall oxygen outlet.

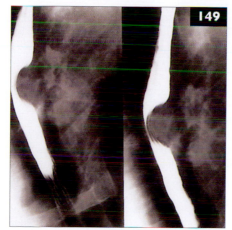

149 Enumerate the types of mediastinal involvement by lung cancer and how they may present. What is the cause of this radiological appearance (**149**)?

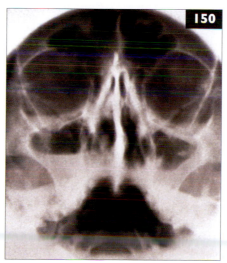

150 i. What is the diagnosis of the condition shown in **150**, and what are the symptoms?
ii. What are the predisposing factors?
iii. What is the relationship between asthma and sinus disease?

149 Mediastinal involvement includes the following:
- Left recurrent laryngeal nerve palsy presents as hoarseness and poor cough. It is due to metastases in the subaortic fossa.
- Superior vena caval obstruction is caused by tumour compression by the right paratracheal lymph nodes.
- Dysphagia can be due to mediastinal lymphadenopathy of the subcarinal modes. A barium swallow will identify the location of the obstruction (shown here).
- Arrhythmias, usually atrial fibrillation, can be caused by direct pericardial invasion by tumour, particularly from the left lower lobe.
- Pericardial effusion – as above, this is due to direct invasion by tumour. Tamponade can ensue with dyspnoea and appropriate physical signs.
- High hemidiaphragm can occur, which is due to phrenic nerve entrapment in the mediastinum.

Horner's syndrome results, usually, from a primary apical tumour extending onto the posterior mediastinal surface and entrapping the sympathetic chain. It is characterized by a small pupil with enophthalmos on the affected side. There is partial ptosis due to paralysis of the sympathetically innervated portion of the orbicularis oculis muscle (Müller's muscle). There is also a unilateral absence of sweating on the face and forehead.

150 i. Paranasal sinusitis. There is bilateral mucosal thickening and air–fluid levels in the maxillary sinuses, worse on the left. Symptoms include headache, pain, and tenderness over the affected sinuses, periorbital swelling in children, nasal congestion and obstruction, purulent nasal secretions, postnasal drainage, cough, sore throat, and purulent sputum. A CT scan of the paranasal sinuses is a very sensitive and specific means of showing sinus disease.

ii. Predisposing factors include acute viral, bacterial, mycoplasmal, or other respiratory tract infections, foreign bodies, nasogastric or nasotracheal tubes, nasal packing, exposures to respiratory tract irritants, and barotrauma associated with flying, swimming, and diving. More longstanding risk factors include allergic rhinitis, nasal polyposis, immunoglobulin deficiencies, AIDS, anatomical disorders, cystic fibrosis, or ciliary dyskinesia syndrome.

iii. Sinusitis is a frequent finding in patients with asthma and can lead to a worsening of asthma. Sinusitis with nasal mucosal congestion and oedema results in decreased humidification and temperature rectification of inhaled air. Sinusitis is associated with postnasal drainage, which can carry bacteria and/or inflammatory material to the lower respiratory tract. Asthma and sinusitis are also linked through a common allergic response pathway or aspirin sensitivity.

151 A 62-year-old male presents with a 2-week history of confusion and headaches. He also has a longstanding history of cough, and an abnormal chest X-ray shows hilar lymphadenopathy. His fundoscopy is shown here (**151**).
i. Describe the appearances of the fundoscopy.
ii. What is the likely diagnosis?
iii. What further investigations should be performed to confirm the diagnosis?

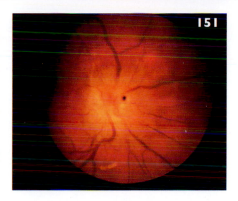

152 i. What is this scan (**152**)?
ii. When does one order this test?
iii. How useful is it?
iv. How often does it change the clinical staging of a lung cancer?

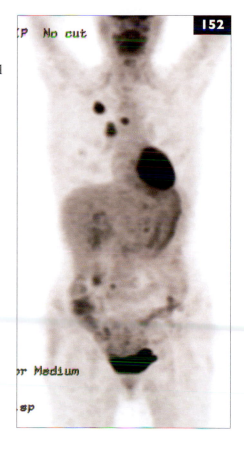

151 i. Fundoscopy shows blurring of the optic disc consistent with papilloedema.
ii. The most likely diagnosis is neurosarcoidosis.
iii. An MRI scan of the brain with gadolinium would show leptomeningeal enhancement and periventricular high-signal lesions on T2-weighted images. A lumbar puncture (after raised intracranial pressure has been excluded) would show lymphocytes and a raised CSF protein level, often greater than 1 g/l. CSF ACE may be raised, and oligoclonal bands should be absent. Serum ACE is also often raised but is not sufficiently sensitive or specific to be useful for diagnosis, although it is commonly used to monitor the disease response to treatment. A CT scan of the chest is required to elucidate the bilateral hilar lymphadenopathy and identify mediastinal nodes and any parenchymal disease. The pathological diagnosis of sarcoid is made from non-caseating granulomas. The thoracic disease may be diagnosed by bronchoscopy, transbronchial biopsies, endoscopic/endobronchial ultrasound, or mediastinoscopy.

An important differential diagnosis is TB, which may also cause bilateral hilar lymphadenopathy and lymphocytic meningitis. CSF findings include lymphocytes and very high protein levels. Although the CSF is usually smear negative for acid-fast bacilli, TB is commonly identified by PCR or culture. TB is characterized by caseating granulomas that are obtained from mediastinal lymph node biopsy, or by identifying or culturing the organism from sputum or lung lavage.

152 i. This is a PET scan using an intravenous tracer of 18-fluoro-deoxyglucose, which is taken up by cells rapidly metabolizing glucose, such as tumours and infections. The more aggressive the tumour, the higher the uptake (standardized uptake value). The PET scan shows the primary tumour uptake and hilar plus right paratracheal node uptake.
ii. This test should follow CT and diagnosis if a tumour appears resectable.
iii. It is extremely useful as it is much superior to CT at identifying hitherto occult lesions. The resolution of PET is limited to lesions greater than 7 mm in size, but it will identify metastatic disease in up to 30% of cases staged by CT scanning alone. PET can give a false-positive result in up to 10% of cases, and apparently positive lesions should be biopsied. False-negative PET is rare and does not need biopsy confirmation. Slow-growing tumours, including alveolar cell carcinoma and carcinoid tumours, can be falsely negative, however. False positives are seen with distal infection, TB, sarcoid, fungal infections, and rheumatoid nodules.
iv. PET changes the staging of the cancer usually by downstaging it, i.e. assigning it a worse stage, in up to 35% of subjects and will save a thoracotomy in up to 20% of individuals as assessed by CT and isotope scanning alone.

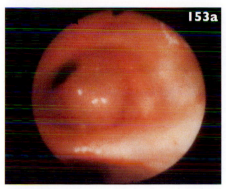
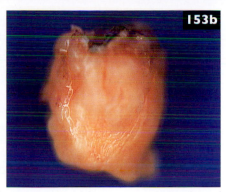

153 This 70-year-old patient has had haemoptysis with recurrent episodes of pneumonia in the left lower lobe for 15 years. A mass (153a, 153b) was seen at bronchoscopy to be partially occluding the left lower lobe and was removed by laser resection. What is the likely diagnosis?

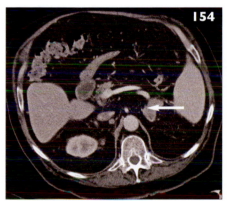
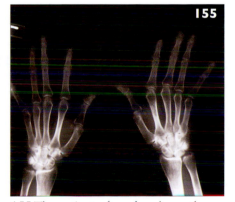

154 i. What does the CT scan (154) show?
ii. Why is this important?
iii. How would you make the diagnosis?

155 The patient whose hands are shown in the radiograph (155) suffers from difficulty swallowing, arthralgias, and a waxy appearance of the skin on her face and distal extremities.
i. What disorder accounts for these abnormalities?
ii. What are the two general types of pulmonary disease associated with this disorder?

153 Given the long history, the polypoid mass is likely to be a benign endobronchial tumour. The majority of these are carcinoid tumours, although they may be locally invasive, and metastases to the hilar lymph nodes may be seen at resection. These tumours show neuroendocrine differentiation, but the carcinoid syndrome is rare in bronchial carcinoids. Other benign bronchial tumours are of mesenchymal origin and include lipomas, leiomyomas, and fibromas. This tumour was a mixed fibrolipoma, and the laser resection line can be seen at the base of the polyp. Rigid bronchoscopy and laser were used because significant haemorrhage may occur with the removal of these tumours, particularly carcinoid tumours.

Endobronchial obstruction should be suspected in cases of recurrent pneumonia, particularly when associated with haemoptysis. Inhaled foreign bodies may cause the same syndrome. Foreign bodies may not be visible on chest radiographs. Other non-malignant causes of endobronchial obstruction include amyloidosis and tracheopathia osteoplastica, a cartilaginous proliferation in the major airways. The latter may be a long-term sequel of amyloidosis. Both of these conditions may be resected using laser if the obstruction is symptomatic.

154 i. The scan shows a left-sided adrenal metastasis with enlargement of the adrenal gland, which is bulky and has lost its triangular shape.
ii. If an adrenal mass is found during the staging of a lung cancer, the concern is that it is a metastasis. One series found that of 330 patients with apparently operable tumours, 7.5% (25) had an adrenal mass, of which eight (2.4) were malignant, i.e. only about 30% of the masses.
iii. Taking into account the information from (ii), either a biopsy should be performed to confirm the nature of the mass, or a PET scan should be undertaken. If the latter is negative, no further investigation if needed, but if it is positive, a biopsy is needed, usually under CT control. Adrenal metastases are found in up to 40% of cases of lung cancer at autopsy.

155 i. Progressive systemic sclerosis (or scleroderma) is a connective tissue disease in which progressive fibrosis and collagen replacement affects multiple organs, including the skin, oesophagus, joints, and lung. The hand radiograph depicts acro-osteolysis or erosion of the distal phalanges. Pulmonary symptoms include dyspnoea and cough.
ii. The most common pulmonary manifestation of systemic sclerosis is fibrosing alveolitis, the pattern of which is indistinguishable from idiopathic pulmonary fibrosis (cryptogenic fibrosing alveolitis). A second, less common pulmonary manifestation is pulmonary hypertension. The severity of the pulmonary hypertension of progressive systemic sclerosis is not predicted by the degree of restrictive interstitial disease.

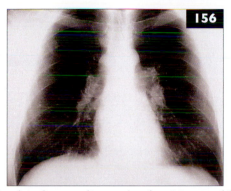

156 Shown (**156**) is the chest radiograph of a 44-year-old male with a non-productive cough for 3 months that resolved after treatment for a postnasal drip. Skin tests were negative for tuberculin and positive for histoplasmin. He recalled no childhood respiratory illnesses and had been raised on a farm in Illinois.
i. What are the radiographic findings?
ii. What is the differential diagnosis?

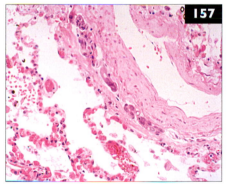

157 i. What does the open lung biopsy in **157** show?
ii. What is its pathogenesis?
iii. What conditions predispose to this appearance?

156 i. The chest radiograph shows hilar and paratracheal adenopathy, and diffusely scattered, small, calcified parenchymal lung nodules. This appearance suggests a remote and now 'healed' disseminated infection.

ii. The differential diagnosis includes previous infection (e.g. varicella, histoplasmosis) or, less likely, sarcoidosis. Miliary TB or disseminated coccidioidomycosis is unlikely to have resolved spontaneously, and transbronchial lung biopsies in the patient failed to demonstrate active peribronchial granulomatous inflammation. Thus, 'old' histoplasmosis is the most likely explanation for these radiographic abnormalities.

Histoplasmosis results from the inhalation of spores of the dimorphic soil fungus *Histoplasma capsulatum*, which is endemic to the central river valleys of North America. Acute infection is often asymptomatic but can occasionally result in a pneumonia-like illness or even ARDS. Parenchymal infiltrates and hilar adenopathy may be seen even in asymptomatic patients. Fibrosis and calcification often accompany the resolution of these infections, and hepatosplenic calcification may also be present. Most patients recover without medical intervention.

Some patients (generally those with underlying lung disease) fail to clear the initial infection and develop chronic pulmonary histoplasmosis, which clinically and radiologically resembles TB. Progressive disseminated histoplasmosis can be life-threatening, especially in patients with defective cell-mediated immunity. This may occur during progressive primary infection but more often results from reactivation in previously infected patients. Both chronic and disseminated histoplasmosis should be treated with amphotericin B, although oral itraconazole may be used in milder cases. Immunocompromised patients require chronic suppressive itraconazole therapy.

157 i. The lymphatic channels next to the large vessel are infiltrated by tumour cells. There is some vascular congestion. Both are typical of lymphangitis carcinomatosa.

ii. Tumour enters the lungs via the pulmonary arteries and embeds in the vessel wall, from where it penetrates into the adjacent lymphatics with subsequent permeation throughout the lung. Some patients only have spread within the vascular tree. A marked reduction in carbon monoxide gas transfer may be demonstrated in these cases of vascular permeation.

iii. The most common tumour that gives rise to this condition is adenocarcinoma; primary sites include breast, stomach, prostate, ovary, endometrium, pancreas, and colon. When these tumours are known to be present, the diagnosis is relatively simple. However, lymphangitis carcinomatosa may be the presenting symptoms of these tumours so the cause of breathlessness may be confused with pulmonary oedema or benign causes of interstitial lung disease until transbronchial or open lung biopsy is performed.

Measurement	Observed maximum	Predicted maximum
Heart rate (beats/min)	162	160
Ventilation (l/min)	55	60
VO_2max (l/min)	1.9	–

158 The data shown in the *Table* were obtained at maximal exercise testing in a 45-year-old male with breathlessness on exertion.
i. What does VO_2max measure, and what parameters are needed to measure it?
ii. Would this patient be capable of performing a job involving packing shelves with lightweight boxes?

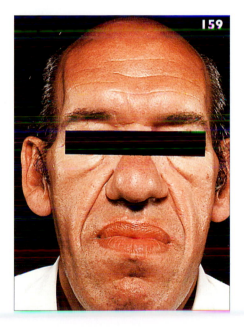

159 i. What is the cause of this patient's OSA?
ii. How would you treat this condition?
iii. How would you make the diagnosis?
iv. If the sleep apnoea is severe, what precaution would you take prior to and after surgery?

158 i. VO_2 measures the amount of oxygen extracted by the tissues during exercise and is directly related to the amount of work performed. VO_2 = cardiac output (Q) x oxygen content difference of arterial and mixed venous blood ($CaO_2 - CvO_2$), or $VO_2 = Q \times (SaO_2 - SvO_2) \times 1.34$.

SvO_2 (the saturation of mixed venous blood) reflects the ability of the exercising muscles to extract oxygen from the blood. VO_2max is defined as the plateau of oxygen uptake where attempting to go beyond that work capacity is associated with increasing ventilation but no increase in cardiac output. This is the point at which the subject has reached maximal aerobic power. Many subjects do not reach this point as it requires considerable effort and determination with unpleasant sensations of breathlessness and muscle soreness. Therefore what is often reported is the maximum VO_2 achieved and not the true VO_2max. VO_2 can be obtained from work performed on a cycle ergometer, treadmill, or even stepping exercise, provided that measures of minute ventilation and mixed expired oxygen and carbon dioxide tensions are available.
ii. To be able to perform heavy physical labour throughout an 8-hr shift, subjects should achieve a VO_2max of >25 ml/kg/min. Subjects whose VO_2max is <15 ml/kg/min would be unable to walk at more than a normal pace. Therefore the result here suggests he should be able to perform his relatively light tasks.

159 i. Acromegaly – there is typical frontal bossing with prominent supraorbital ridges, prognathism, coarse skin, and thickened lips. Another endocrinological cause of OSA is myxoedema.
ii. Transsphenoidal removal of the pituitary gland. Octreotide, which is a somatostatin analogue, has also been reported to improve OSA in some patients with acromegaly. Despite successful surgery, most acromegalic patients continue to have significant sleep apnoea, which requires treatment with nasal CPAP.
iii. OSA is likely to be severe as the tongue is enlarged in this condition, and oropharyngeal blockage during sleep likely to be severe. Therefore a simple screening sleep test with an oximeter will record successive dips of SaO_2 throughout sleep.
iv. The patient should be put on nasal CPAP before and immediately after surgery, even if the surgery is potentially curative. This is because anaesthesia and opiates can cause a further reduction in upper airway tone and a suppression of the arousal response to obstruction. Once the patient has recovered from the surgery, a repeat sleep study should check whether there is still significant OSA.

Test	Range	Result	% Predicted
FEV$_1$ (l)	1.79–2.42	1.1	52
FVC (l)	2.42–3.26	1.25	44
FEV$_1$/FVC (%)	70–84	89	119
TLC (l)	4.4–5.96	3.5	60
RV (l)	1.62–2.19	1.8	95
DL$_{CO}$ (mmol/ min/kPa)	6.15–8.31	2.75	38
Alveolar volume (l)		2.0	
K$_{CO}$ (mmol/ min/kPa/l)	1.4–1.9	1.35	82

160 A 28-year-old male is wheelchair bound and presents with morning headaches. His lung function tests are shown in the *Table*.
i. What type of underlying condition does he have?
ii. Explain the lung function results.
iii. What other lung function tests may be useful?

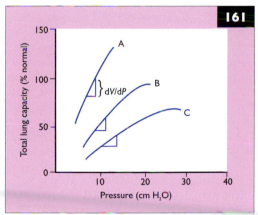

161 The figure (**161**) shows three pressure–volume curves of the lung and also lung compliance (dV/dP).
i. Which is the normal curve, and which are those of disease?
ii. Which types of disease do the abnormal curves (a, b, or c) depict and why?

160 i. Neuromuscular disorder, e.g. myotonic dystrophy causing respiratory muscle weakness. Morning headaches may be due to hypercapnia and suggest type II respiratory failure.

ii. Lung function tests demonstrate a restrictive FEV_1/FVC ratio with a reduced TLC. The DL_{CO} is significantly reduced at 38% predicted, but when corrected for the alveolar volume the K_{CO} is preserved. This implies a chest wall or muscle abnormality (rather than a parenchymal abnormality, in which the K_{CO} would also be reduced). The RV may be normal or even increased in severe respiratory muscle weakness.

iii. Other tests may be useful in establishing a diagnosis of respiratory muscle weakness. The fall in VC between the upright and supine positions has been used to assess diaphragmatic weakness and is a more sensitive indicator of respiratory muscle weakness than upright measures of VC and TLC. Normally, there is less than a 10% drop in VC when changing from the upright to the supine position. With bilateral diaphragm paralysis or weakness, VC may be reduced by more than 30% in the supine position.

Maximal inspiratory and expiratory pressures are also abnormal in respiratory muscle weakness. Generalized neuromuscular weakness reduces both maximum inspiratory and maximum expiratory pressure, whereas isolated involvement of the diaphragm, such as with idiopathic diaphragm paralysis or the early stages of amyotrophic lateral sclerosis, may reduce only maximum inspiratory pressure. The sniff test is another test of global respiratory muscle function.

161 i. The normal curve is curve B. The lung is most compliant at an FRC that is approximately at 40% that of TLC in normal individuals. This is the most compliant part of the pressure–volume curve, where breathing in occurs with least effort for the greatest expansion.

ii. Curve A is from a patient with emphysema. The loss of elastic recoil caused by the destructive emphysema means that the maximum recoil pressure of the lung (at TLC) is reduced compared with normal. Therefore the lung remains more expanded than normal at any given lung volume owing to its poor recoil pressures. In addition, the lung is more compliant, so breathing in at FRC (at a greater lung volume than normal) remains easy, but expiration will be more difficult due to the ready collapsibility of the lungs.

Curve C is from a patient with interstitial lung disease. The lung is less compliant and stiffer due to the increased intrinsic fibrosis. Owing to the loss of compliance, inspiration, even at FRC, is harder than normal, increasing the work of breathing. The total elastic recoil pressure at TLC is greater than normal. These stiff, inelastic lungs suffer pneumotharaces more readily than normal lungs, and any such pneumothorax is slow to heal because of the high elastic recoil pressures encouraging the lung to collapse.

162 i. Describe the appearances of these hands (**162**).
ii. What are the pulmonary manifestations of this disease?

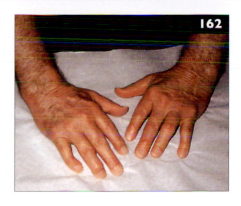

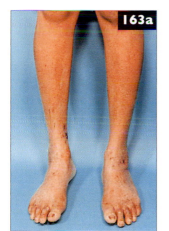

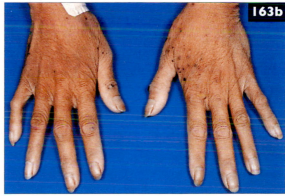

163 This 52-year-old male presented with this painless rash on his ankles (**163a**) and wrists (**163b**). The chest radiograph was abnormal.
i. Describe the rash.
ii. What pulmonary conditions are associated with this type of rash?

Pulmonary manifestations of rheumatoid arthritis

Pleurisy
Pleural thickening
Pleural effusion
• Exudate
• High cholesterol
• Low glucose <1.5 mmol/l, low pH <7.2
• Low C3 and C4; positive rheumatoid factor
Rheumatoid nodules
• Typically subpleural distribution
• May rupture into the pleural space, causing pneumothorax and bronchopleural fistula

Usual interstitial pneumonitis
Non-specific interstitial pneumonitis
Organizing pneumonia
Bronchiectasis
BO
Mediastinal lymphadenopathy
Cricoarytenoid arthritis
Rheumatoid nodules of the larynx

---

162 i. The hands demonstrate the swelling of the metacarpophalangeal joints and ulnar deviation characteristic of rheumatoid arthritis.
ii. The pulmonary manifestations are listed in the *Box*.

163 i. The patient has a typical vasculitic rash with small haemorrhagic lesions on his forearms and shins.
ii. Vasculitis can affect the lungs as part of a systemic condition. The more common conditions include:
• Wegener's granulomatosis.
• Allergic granulomatosis and angiitis (Churg–Strauss syndrome). This comprises asthma, hypereosinophilia with eosinophilic infiltrates, vasculitis, and granulomas in various organs. It can be controlled by oral steroids, but the vasculitis can be life-threatening. The condition usually begins with asthma at about 35 years of age, and is of equal sex incidence; the vasculitis follows some years later. Upper airway lesions, usually as allergic rhinitis, are common. The ANCA test, predominantly perinuclear ANCA, is positive in 50% of patients.
• Polyarteritis nodosa, which affects medium-sized arteries, while Churg–Strauss syndrome affects small ones. There is usually no history of allergic illness in polyarteritis nodosa, and pulmonary involvement is not common. Pulmonary involvement includes asthma, pulmonary infiltrates, fibrosis, and effusions. The cytoplasmic ANCA test is negative.

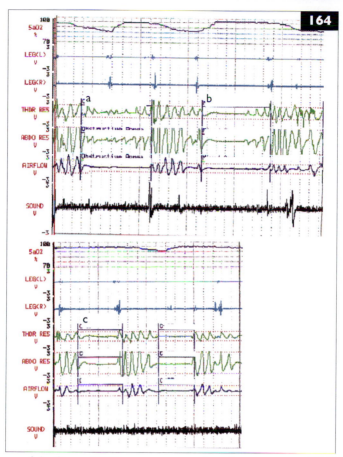

164 Parts **a–c** of the figure (**164**) are segments of a polysomnogram [LEG(R)(L), leg movement; THOR RES, ABDO RES, thoracic and abdominal movement]. Which of these shows?:

i. Obstructive apnoea.

ii. Central apnoea.

iii. Mixed apnoea.

165 What is the ILO (International Labour Office) classification for pneumoconiosis?

164 i. Obstructive apnoeas (**164a**) are characterized by a cessation of airflow with continued evidence of respiratory effort on the chest and abdominal traces, often in a paradoxical fashion. SaO_2 decreases during these episodes, periodically reaching a nadir at the end of or just after the reinitiation of airflow.

ii. Central apnoeas (**164c**) result in a cessation of airflow with no evidence of respiratory effort on the chest and abdominal traces. This event was terminated by an EEG arousal.

iii. Mixed apnoeas (**164b**), a variant of OSA, consist of a central event followed by an obstructive portion (respiratory effort begins before airflow does).

165 It is a method of grading the size of opacities on chest radiography due to pneumoconiosis, primarily for epidemiological reporting. The number of opacities correlates with the quantity of dust in the lungs. The opacities may be the dust itself or the consequent fibrosis. There is a broad division between opacities of up to 1 cm (simple pneumoconiosis), and those over 1 cm diameter (complicated pneumoconiosis, or progressive massive fibrosis). Progressive massive fibrosis arises on a background of simple pneumoconiosis.

Profusion gives an estimate of the density of the nodules, and is determined by comparison with a set of standardized radiographs (*Table*). Each profusion category can be subdivided into three, to give a 12-point scale; p nodules are mostly seen in coal-worker's pneumoconiosis, whereas r nodules are associated with silicosis.

Lung function changes with simple coal-worker's pneumoconiosis are usually minimal and often overshadowed by the effects of cigarette smoking, although coal dust does contribute to the development of emphysema. Radiographic changes do not progress after the miner leaves the coal face with simple pneumoconiosis, but they can occur with progressive massive fibrosis. With silica exposure, simple changes may, however, progress despite removal from the offending agent. Those developing progressive massive fibrosis have usually been exposed to a high dust burden. Progressive hypoxaemia usually occurs. It is important to exclude other causes of large irregular opacities such as tumours and infection.

Simple			
Nodule size	Rounded nodules	Irregular nodules	Profusion of nodules
<1.5 mm	p	s	0, 1, 2 or 3
1.5–3 mm	q	t	0, 1, 2 or 3
3–10 mm	r	u	0, 1, 2 or 3

Complicated	
Nodule size	Category
1–5 cm, or several with combined diameter up to 5 cm	A
Between A and B	B
One or more with combined area >1/3 of lung field	C

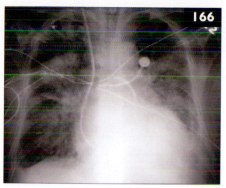

166 The abnormalities seen on the chest radiograph (**166**) developed suddenly in a patient with a history of recent intravenous drug use.
i. What is the differential diagnosis?
ii. How might information obtained from the pulmonary artery catheter affect the differential diagnosis?
iii. How might the history of heroin use relate to the abnormalities shown?

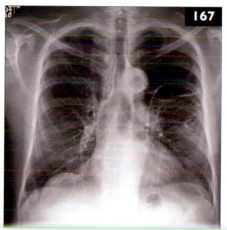

167 This is the chest X-ray (**167**) of a 62-year-man with a 3-year history of slowly progressive exertional dyspnoea. He has a 30 pack–year history of smoking cigarettes.
i. What does the chest X-ray show?
ii. What investigations are necessary?
iii. What non-medical interventions are possible to improve this patient's dyspnoea?

166 i. The differential diagnosis of acute interstitial infiltrates can be divided into cardiogenic causes and conditions resulting in increased vascular permeability. Cardiogenic causes include congestive heart failure, myocardial infarction or coronary insufficiency, acute valvular heart disease, severe volume overload, and acute diastolic dysfunction. Increased permeability can result from near-drowning, heroin or other drug overdose, sepsis, chest trauma, burns, or exposure to toxic gases. The oedema that develops at high altitude may result from abnormalities in both intravascular pressure and permeability.

ii. A pulmonary artery catheter allows measurement of the pulmonary arterial occlusion (wedge) pressure as a reflection of the left ventricular preload and/or the intravascular hydrostatic pressure in the pulmonary capillaries (ignoring the effects of possible venoconstriction) and can frequently separate cardiac from permeability problems. A wedge pressure of >18 cmH_2O suggests cardiac abnormalities.

iii. As stated above, heroin and other opiate drugs – illicit as well as conventional use – can cause acute non-cardiogenic pulmonary oedema. Intravenous drugs are also associated with alterations in consciousness leading to widespread aspiration, to acute myocardial dysfunction (cocaine), or to valvular incompetence (acute bacterial endocarditis).

167 i. The chest X-ray shows a large left upper zone thin-walled cyst suggestive of a bulla. The main and important differential diagnosis is tethered pneumothorax – it is vital that bullae are not mistaken for a tethered pneumothorax as the insertion of a chest drain into a bulla will create a bronchopleural fistula that will require surgical intervention and can be potentially fatal. As in this case, bullae often do not have a well-defined medial edge, whereas a pneumothorax should always have a clearly defined edge.

ii. CT scanning is useful to characterize the number, size, and location of the bullae, and should be used to differentiate between a tethered pneumothorax and bullae if there is any doubt *before* chest drain insertion. In this patient, the CT scan demonstrated that although there is a particularly large bulla in the left upper lobe, there are in addition several other bullae in both lungs. Lung function testing is necessary to identify the severity of disease and as a baseline to judge the success of any therapeutic interventions. Basal bullae are associated with α_1-antitrypsin deficiency.

iii. Pulmonary rehabilitation can help to improve a patient's exercise tolerance. Bullectomy can improve lung function by allowing compressed relatively normal lung to re-expand and needs to be considered, especially if the remaining lung is relatively normal with little emphysema present.

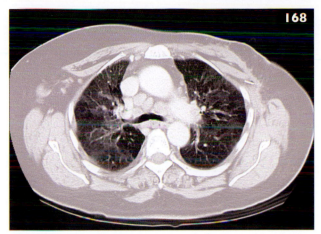

168 This 35-year-old female has a 4-month history of wheeze, cough, and exertional breathlessness. She has kept parakeets for the past 4 years. Auscultation of the chest reveals inspiratory crackles. Her HRCT is shown (**168**).
i. Describe the appearances and their differential diagnoses.
ii. How may the diagnosis be confirmed?

169 A 69-year-old male underwent a right upper lobectomy a year ago for an adenocarcinoma of the lung. He now presents with a 3-week history of frontal headaches and a 2-day history of dysphasia.
i. What is the likely diagnosis?
ii. How common is this at the diagnosis of the primary lung cancer and as a metastatic manifestation?
iii. What are the treatment options?

168 i. The HRCT shows mosaic attenuation. The mosaic attenuation pattern may represent patchy interstitial disease, small airways disease, or occlusive vascular disease. In this case, air trapping due to small airways obstruction causes focal areas of decreased attenuation, which are enhanced by using expiratory-phase images. Mosaic attenuation may also be produced by interstitial ground-glass opacity, where the areas of high attenuation represent the interstitial process and areas of low attenuation the normal lung.

ii. The clinical scenario is highly suggestive of 'bird-fancier's lung' – a subacute hypersensitivity pneumonitis (EAA) that predominantly affects the upper zones. If left untreated, the condition may progress to chronic fibrosis. Avian precipitins are positive. Lung biopsy (transbronchial via bronchoscopy or surgical) will demonstrate non-caseating granulomas in a peribronchial distribution. Avoidance of the precipitating antigen results in improvement of the symptoms and aids the diagnosis.

169 i. The patient has developed cerebral metastases. The CT scan (**169**) showed multiple lesions. These typically show ring enhancement after intravenous contrast, and a surrounding darker area of cerebral oedema.

ii. Cerebral metastases occur most commonly in small-cell and adenocarcinoma, and least with squamous cell carcinoma. They are most commonly associated with upper lobe tumours. The typical symptoms are many but most commonly headache, vomiting, visual field loss, speech disorders, cranial nerve signs, fits, and long tract abnormalities. Posterior fossa metastases are also common, causing giddiness or failure to heel–toe walk if the lesion is in the midline of the posterior fossa. Cerebral metastases occur in about 5% of individuals at the time of diagnosis of lung cancer, and this is the first site of relapse in up to 20% of cases, with 50% having brain metastases at autopsy.

iii. Initial treatment is with steroids. A good response will be due to clearing of the cerebral oedema. Radiotherapy may maintain this improvement, but if there is little response to steroids, radiotherapy will not usually be very effective. The median survival after developing brain metastases is 2–4 months. Prophylactic whole-brain radiotherapy is given to patients with small-cell disease with a complete response to

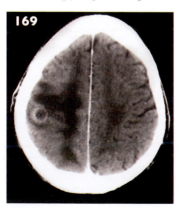

chemotherapy. This prevents brain relapse and improves median survival by a few months. Occasional patients with a single brain metastasis on MRI (a better investigation than CT) may undergo resection of the primary tumour followed by cerebral metastatectomy, with a 5-year survival of about 25% in very small series.

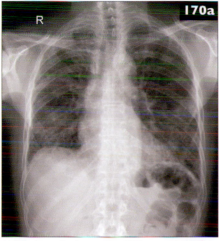

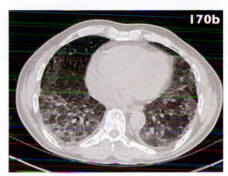

170 A 47-year-old male was given chemotherapy for acute lymphoblastic leukaemia. He developed persistent cough and increasingly severe dyspnoea over a 6-week period; his chest X-ray (170a) and thoracic CT scan (170b) are shown. He was apyrexial, markedly dyspnoeic on exertion, with fine bilateral crepitations to both mid-zones and a resting saturation of 93% on air.

i. What does the CT scan show?
ii. What is the likely cause of this radiological appearance?
iii. What lung function abnormalities would be expected?

171 i. What is the differential diagnosis of daytime hypersomnolence?
ii. How would the history help in differentiating these diagnoses?

172 A young male presented to the Accident & Emergency department complaining of left chest pain and breathlessness after a kick to the left side of the body.
i. What does the chest radiograph (172) show?
ii. What is the differential diagnosis and what surgical treatment should be offered?

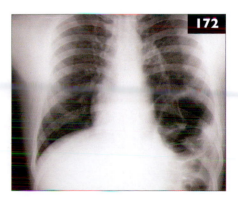

170 i. The CT scan shows widespread ground-glass infiltrations in both lungs and marked subpleural changes suggestive of pulmonary fibrosis.

ii. The likely diagnosis is a drug reaction causing a pneumonitis and pulmonary fibrosis. These can occur after treatment with a wide range of chemotherapy agents. The onset varies but is usually within a few weeks of treatment, and the reaction can be severe enough to cause respiratory failure and death. As well as withdrawing the causative agent, oral corticosteroids are frequently used to try to reverse the lung damage, or at least reduce its progression.

iii. Lung function tests will show a restrictive defect, small lung volumes, and a marked impairment of gas transfer. The patient often destaurates markedly on exercise even if the resting oxygen saturations are normal.

171 i. The differential diagnosis includes intrinsic causes such as OSA, narcolepsy, idiopathic hypersomnia, post-traumatic hypersomnia, periodic movements of the legs/restless sleep, and extrinsic causes such as poor 'sleep hygiene', insufficient sleep, hypnotic/sedative abuse, and alcohol abuse.

ii. In OSA, there is a history of a steady progression of symptoms, often over many years. Initially there is snoring, which becomes more pronounced, turning into periods of apnoea and restlessness that become more numerous and prolonged. This is noted by the partner rather than the patient. The condition develops fully by middle age, is more common in males, and is associated with weight gain, increased alcohol intake, and night sedation. In classical narcolepsy, there is a history of cataplexy and at least one of the other three symptoms: sleepiness, sleep paralysis, and hypnagogic hallucinations. In periodic leg movement, there is an irresistible urge to move the legs, causing insomnia and sleep disruption. In post-traumatic hypersomnia, there is a history of preceding head injury, stroke, or brain surgery.

172 i. The left hemithorax contains gas-filled loops of intestine.

ii. The differential diagnosis includes a raised hemidiaphragm, eventration of the diaphragm, congenital diaphragmatic hernia, and, given the history of trauma, traumatic rupture of the diaphragm.

Eventration of the diaphragm results from paralysis, hypoplasia, or atrophy of the muscle fibres. It can be difficult to diagnose even on CT scan and is often confirmed only at surgery. The aim of surgery in eventration is to incise the thinned-out diaphragmatic leaf and to repair the diaphragm by imbricating one layer over the other. In diaphragmatic hernia or traumatic rupture, the diaphragm is repaired either by direct suture or by the placement of a 'patch' (marlex mesh) across the defect.

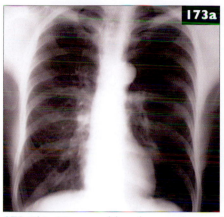
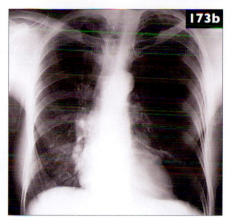

173 This 30-year-old male complains of mild exertional dyspnoea.
i. What condition is suggested by the chest radiographs on inspiration (**173a**) and expiration (**173b**), and what is the possible aetiology?
ii. What else should the condition be distinguished from?

174 i. Approximately what percentage of chronic cigarette smokers develop airflow limitation?
ii. What are the benefits of smoking cessation in terms of pulmonary function?
iii. What strategies are available for aiding smoking cessation?

175 i. Describe the appearances in this chest radiograph (**175**) from a male with a long history of gastrointestinal symptoms.
ii. What are the most likely causative organisms?
iii. What is the treatment of choice?

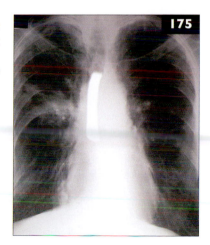

173 i. The radiographic finding of a unilateral radiolucent lung was described by Macleod and is also known as Swyer–James syndrome. The syndrome is ascribed to neonatal or early childhood BO. The lung is usually otherwise normal and well preserved, but with small pulmonary vessels. Large air spaces can develop, with poor ventilation of the affected lung, which may remain fully inflated on an expiratory film (**173b**). The prognosis is good.

ii. Other causes of a radiolucent appearance to a lung include congenital absence of the chest wall muscles or mastectomy, obstruction to a pulmonary artery by embolus or tumour, compression of the pulmonary artery by tumour or nodes, and congenital abnormalities. The partial obstruction of a main bronchus by a tumour or a foreign body can occasionally produce unilateral hyperlucency.

174 i. Only approximately 15% of smokers develop airflow limitation. Accordingly, other unknown factors must contribute to this problem (e.g. genetic susceptibility such as other yet to be determined protease abnormalities).

ii. The rate of decline in FEV_1 in continuing smokers (around 30–140 ml/year) is greater than that of ex-smokers in which the rate approaches that of non-smokers (30 ml/year). Thus, smoking cessation can reduce the rate of loss of lung function and thereby to a large extent determine the patient's subsequent clinical course. Clearly, much depends on the habitual activity of the subject as to when he or she presents. A manual worker may notice dyspnoea before a sedentary person. Unfortunately, dyspnoea occurs with when a gross deterioration in lung function has already occurred in the majority of susceptible smokers.

iii. Smoking cessation clinics and hypnotherapy have generally been unsuccessful. Transdermal nicotine patches, and to a lesser extent nicotine gum, seem valuable. The nicotine dose (5, 10, or 20 mg per patch) can be titrated to the patient's level of addiction. The patches should not be worn overnight. Just advising the patient not to smoke should always be offered.

175 i. The chest radiograph shows patchy shadowing in the right mid to upper zone. In the upper mediastinum, the oesophagus is outlined by a column of barium, the appearances therefore suggesting oesophageal obstruction and aspiration pneumonia.

ii. The most likely causative organisms would be normal oropharyngeal commensal organisms, which are typically anaerobes such a *Bacteroides* or *Peptostreptococcus*. If the patient had spent more than 4 days in hospital before aspiration occurred, Gram-negative enterobacteria would also need to be considered.

iii. The treatment of choice for anaerobic lung infections is either a combination of penicillin plus metronidazole, co-amoxiclav, or alternatively clindamycin. The oesophageal obstruction should also be treated.

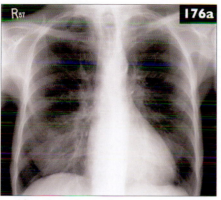

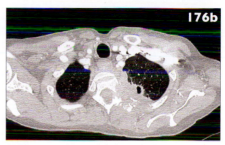

176 A 76-year-old female has seen her GP, a physiotherapist, and a rheumatologist for her now 8-month history of pain and numbness in her left inner arm and hand, with weakness and wasting of the small muscles of her hand. Her chest radiograph (176a) and CT scan (176b) are shown.
i. What is the diagnosis, and why has it taken so long?
ii. What are the treatment options and outcomes?

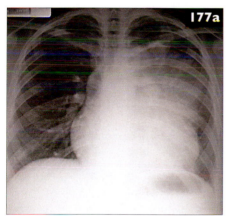

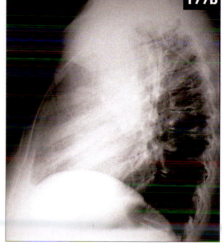

177 This 22-year-old female presented with non-specific malaise and an irritating cough for which her GP arranged a chest radiograph (177a). A lateral XRC (177b) was then performed.
i. What abnormalities are present?
ii. What diagnoses are possible?
iii. How might a diagnosis be achieved?

176 i. The patient has a Pancoast or superior sulcus tumour. The radiograph (**176a**) shows opacification of the left apex with erosion of the medial portion of the left third rib due to a squamous cell or adenocarcinoma. The tumour is asymptomatic until it causes pain by erosion of the posterior third of the second and/or third ribs. It will then invade the brachial plexus, causing TI and C8 nerve root pains that are often thought to be from disease in the shoulder. Wasting and weakness will occur after several months. Horner's syndrome will also occur with more central extension.

The CT scan (**176b**) shows the mass in the posterior part of the left upper lobe with erosion through the rib, extending into the vertebral body and pedicle, and almost encroaching into the spinal canal.

ii. Treatment is usually with radiotherapy, although local recurrence with increasing pain is common and a major management problem. Recently, a combination of preoperative radiotherapy to less advanced cases has been followed by resection. There should be no nodal involvement. This approach in small series has a 5-year survival of 25–35%. In most cases, treatment is palliative with radiotherapy, chemotherapy, and then pain control.

177 i. There is a huge smooth mediastinal mass located in the anterior compartment. Note that the trachea is not deviated laterally despite the left-sided preponderance of the mass, suggesting an anterior origin from the plain chest film. Airway obstruction or even superior vena caval compression may occur.

ii. These appearances could be present with a variety of rapidly growing malignancies, but in a female of this age group, a lymphoma would be a high probability. Other possibilities include a germ cell tumour (in a male), a thymic carcinoma, a primary sarcoma, and metastatic choriocarcinoma. In 90% of adult cases of mediastinal lymphoma, nodular sclerosing Hodgkin's lymphoma is diagnosed (as in this case); 75% of Hodgkin's patients have mediastinal involvement.

iii. Approximately half of the patients with a mediastinal lymphomatous mass have nodes palpable in the neck, and excisional biopsy of one of these would be the least invasive method of getting a tissue sample. If cervical nodes are not present, a CT-guided core biopsy can be performed. Anterior mediastinotomy offers a good way of obtaining a larger specimen. A right- or left-sided biopsy is performed depending on the direction of enlargement of the mass. Mediastinoscopy would be quite impossible and dangerous in a case such as this but can be helpful in providing a diagnosis in patients with modest mediastinal lymphadenopathy.

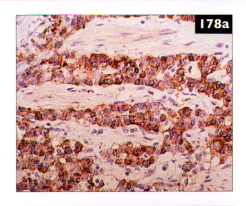

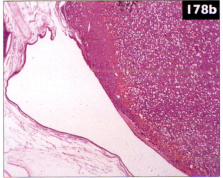

178 i. What stain has been employed on this endobronchial biopsy (**178a, 178b**)?
ii. Is this positive staining specific for this condition?
iii. Are these tumours usually confined to the bronchial lumen?

179 What are the therapeutic options for OSA?

178 i. The histological features of islands and ribbons of cells with uniform nuclei and cytoplasm are consistent with a carcinoid tumour, and the stain chromogranin has been used to verify the neuroendocrine nature of this tumour (**178a**). Other stains that could have been used for this purpose include neurone-specific enolase and synaptophysin.

ii. The stain is specific for cells of neuroendocrine origin; however, other lung tumours of neuroendocrine origin, including small-cell carcinoma and atypical carcinoids, will also be positive for neuroendocrine staining. Therefore the stain is not specific for carcinoid tumours. Indeed, some non-small-cell tumours may have neuroendocrine components. These stains must therefore be employed along with light microscopy, as well as electron microscopy in more difficult cases.

iii. Carcinoid tumours often infiltrate the bronchial wall, and the part of the tumour visible on bronchoscopy may be the 'tip of the iceberg'. **178b** shows the tumour bulging into the bronchial lumen and deforming it. These tumours also tend to be highly vascular and, if suspected by their macroscopic appearance, are preferably biopsied using rigid bronchoscopy.

179 Simple advice for patients with mild-to-moderate OSA includes sleeping on their side, not drinking alcohol after 6 pm, not taking sedatives, losing weight, stopping smoking, and keeping the nose as clear as possible.

The medical treatment of choice is nasal CPAP breathing. This is successful in patients with severe symptoms, who gain considerable and rapid relief and show an improvement in well-being. However, in those with mild OSA, a mandibular advancement splint is effective and may have a higher rate of compliance than CPAP. All patients should receive advise on weight loss and see a trained, interested dietitian.

Surgical treatments include:
• Tonsillectomy and adenoidectomy, especially in children with enlarged tonsils and adenoids, which can cause OSA.
• Uvulopalatopharyngoplasty.
• Nasal surgery: this is generally not useful except in a few individuals who benefit from anterior nasal reconstruction, septal straightening, and polyp removal.
• Maxillary and/or mandibular advancement, a major operation bringing forward the mandible and the maxilla to preserve alignment of the teeth. This is only appropriate if there is a considerable degree of retrognathia with a very narrow retroglossal space and if the patient is unable to tolerate nasal CPAP.
• Tracheostomy: this was used before the availability of nasal CPAP. The tracheostomy is kept closed during the day and open at night.
• Weight loss by gastric surgery: gastric banding and gastrojejunal bypass surgery have become popular in some centres.

Test	Predicted	Range	Result	% predicted
FEV$_1$ (l)	2.10	1.79–2.42	2.10	100
FVC (l)	2.84	2.42–3.26	2.50	88
FEV$_1$ (%)	73	62–84	83	115
FRC (l)	3.00	2.55–3.45	2.42	81
TLC (l)	5.18	4.40–5.96	4.32	83
VC (l)	2.84	2.41–3.26	2.44	86
RV (l)	1.90	1.62–2.19	1.88	99
DL$_{CO}$ (mmol/min/kPa)*	7.23	6.15–8.31	3.48	48
VA†(l)	–	–	3.73	–
K$_{CO}$ (mmol/min/kPa/l)**	1.65	1.40–1.90	0.93	56

*DL$_{CO}$ = transfer factor.   **K$_{CO}$ = transfer coefficient in DL$_{CO}$/VA.
† VA = alveolar volume.

180 These lung function tests (*Table*) are from a 42-year-old female with progressive systemic sclerosis. The chest and cardiac examination were normal, as was the chest radiograph. What is the pathogenesis of the abnormality?

181 A 55-year-old female becomes confused 24 hr after open cholecystectomy. She is obese and has been given high-flow oxygen via a Hudson mask at 8 l/min. Her PaO_2 is 8 kPa, her $PaCO_2$ is 12 kPa, and her blood pH is 7.32.
i. What is happening and why?
ii. How would you treat her?

182 A 30-year-old female presented to the neurologists with diplopia and difficulty swallowing. **182** shows her chest X-ray.
i. What test needs to be performed regularly?
ii. How would the patient's lung function be affected by lying down?
iii. What are the blood gases likely to show?

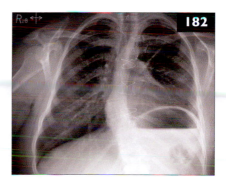

180 Reduction of gas transfer is often the earliest abnormality seen on pulmonary function tests in these patients, and may be due to pulmonary vascular disease or fibrosing alveolitis. The preservation of lung volumes here suggests pulmonary vascular disease. Small pulmonary arteries and arterioles become narrowed due to marked intimal thickening by myxomatous connective tissue. Sequelae are pulmonary hypertension, which may improve with nifedipine if detected early, and eventually cor pulmonale. Pulmonary vascular effects and fibrotic pulmonary disease can occur independently, but often the two pathologies are combined.

181 i. She has type II respiratory failure. She is obese, which will per se cause reduced lung volumes and, when lying flat, a high closing volume and poor gas exchange with hypoxia. She has responded poorly to 40% FiO_2, suggesting a V/Q mismatch. In addition, she is hypoventilating, causing an elevation of $PaCO_2$. This elevation, together with her hypoxaemia, will cause her confusion. She probably also has postoperative abdominal pain, which will further restrict her ventilation. In addition, she may also be on respiratory-suppressive analgesia, which will further compound the problem and add to the hypoventilation.
ii. Treatment should include sitting the patient as upright as possible. Physiotherapy to increase basal expansion and the expectoration of secretions will also be of benefit. If the patient fails to respond to this, assisted ventilation will be required with BiPAP non-invasive ventilation. This, together with adequate analgesia but not using drugs that depress the respiratory centre, will allow BiPAP to be withdrawn after some hours.

182 i. This patient has myasthenia gravis leading to weakness of her ocular and bulbar muscles, and also affecting her respiratory muscles. The chest X-ray shows a unilaterally raised hemidiaphragm with some secondary basal atelectasis. Regular spirometry is necessary to ensure that she does not develop respiratory failure; the spirometry will show a restrictive defect. The chest X-ray is not adequate for assessing diaphragmatic function, and physiological tests are required.
ii. As both hemidiaphragms are likely to be weakened, the abdominal contents will press up into the thoracic cavity on lying down and cause increased dyspnoea and a reduction in the patient's spirometry. For similar reasons, a classical presentation of diaphragmatic palsies is dyspnoea mainly occurring during swimming. The change between the lying and standing FVC can be up to 40%, compared with 10% with normal function.
iii. The blood gases may show type 2 respiratory failure, i.e. increased $PaCO_2$ with a small decrease in the PaO_2, and this is increasingly likely once the FVC falls below 1 litre.

183 i. Describe this chest X-ray (**183**) of a 32-year-old lady with exertional breathlessness.
ii. What is the diagnosis?
iii. What are the possible aetiologies?
iv. What treatments are available?

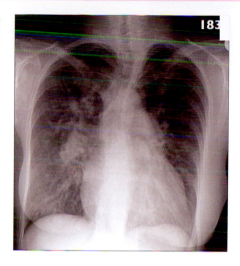

184 This healthy 35-year-old smoker had this X-ray (**184**) at a routine examination.
i. What is the provisional diagnosis?
ii. What is the radiographic stage of the disease, and what investigations would you perform for confirmation?
iii. What is the differential diagnosis?

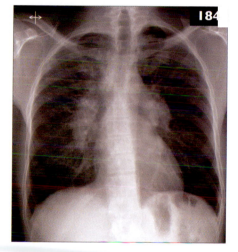

183 i. The chest X-ray shows prominent pulmonary arteries and cardiomegaly.
ii. This is consistent with pulmonary hypertension.
iii. Causes of secondary hypertension can be divided according to their aetiology. When no cause is evident, the condition is called primary pulmonary hypertension, and it more commonly affects younger women. Causes of secondary hypertension include:
- Chronic respiratory disease (which causes hypoxic vasoconstriction), e.g. COPD, sleep apnoea, interstitial lung disease.
- Intrinsic pulmonary vascular pathology, e.g. chronic pulmonary emboli, collagen vascular diseases especially scleroderma, HIV infection, sickle cell disease, amphetamines.
- Cardiac disorders, e.g. mitral valve disease, left ventricular dysfunction, atrial and ventricular septal defects.

iv. Treatments are tailored to the underlying cause. If no cause is identified, effective treatments are limited. Anticoagulation with warfarin may offer some survival benefit. Bosentan (an endothelin antagonist) improves 6-min walk times. Inhaled or intravenous infusions of prostaglandins may also improve symptoms.

184 i. The chest X-ray shows bilaterally and symmetrically enlarged hilar nodes, together with mediastinal nodal enlargement. The lung fields show mid and upper zone infiltrative, and nodular shadowing with no volume loss. The likely diagnosis is sarcoid.
ii. The stage is II. Stage I is hilar adenopathy alone; stage II is bilateral hilar lymphadenopathy with pulmonary infiltration; and stage III is pulmonary infiltration, often with signs of predominant upper lobe fibrosis and volume loss, with resolution of the bilateral hilar lymphadenopathy. If the patient is well and the chest X-ray changes are typical, an elevated serum ACE can suffice for confirmation of the diagnosis. However, to obtain a histological diagnosis, bronchoscopy with transbronchial lung biopsy will reveal non-caseating granulomas in 70–80% of cases. A liver biopsy will furnish a similar yield.
iii. The differential diagnosis is between sarcoid, lymphoma, and TB. For the latter, a biopsy is essential and should be taken if there is any doubt, i.e. if the nodes appear asymmetrical or the patient has relevant symptoms. However, mediastinal node biopsy will be required, and this can now best be done via an endoscopic ultrasound-guided transoesophageal core nodal biopsy.

185 A 50-year-old diabetic male smoker presented with malaise, weight loss, and a persistent cough despite treatment with 7 days of amoxicillin. This is his chest X-ray 3 months after his initial presentation, which is largely unchanged compared with the presentation chest X-ray.
i. What does the chest radiograph show?
ii. What are the possible causes of this radiological appearance?
iii. How should this patient be investigated?

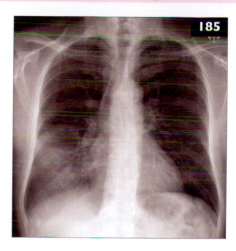

186 A 45-year-old female was found to have this abnormal chest X-ray (**186**) during investigations for an unrelated neurological problem. She had no respiratory symptoms, and apart from her neurological problem she was otherwise well.
i. Describe the abnormality seen.
ii. What are the possible causes?
iii. What investigations are necessary?

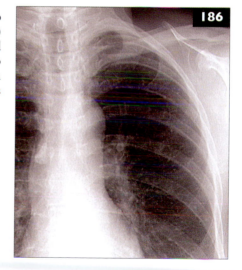

185 i. The chest radiographs X-ray shows persisting right lower zone consolidation over several months.

ii. Persisting consolidation can be due to a subacute infection that has not been treated effectively, such as TB or infection with non-tuberculosis mycobacteria, and the rarer infectious diseases such as actinomycocis or nocardiasis. In addition, non-infective causes need to be considered, including bronchial obstruction due to a tumour or foreign body, or a malignancy that mimics consolidation such as alveolar cell carcinoma or lymphoma.

iii. The patient needs repeated sputum sent for microscopy and culture for conventional and mycobacterial pathogens as well as cytological evaluation, a CT scan of the chest, and bronchoscopy to both exclude an obstructive lesion and obtain a bronchial wash or lavage for culture and cytology. In this patient, bronchoscopy was macroscopically normal, but *Actinomyces* were identified in the bronchial washings. Actinomycosis causes subacute infections presenting as focal areas of consolidation that can extend through the chest wall. Diagnosis is either by culture, requiring prolonged anaerobic culture, or by microscopy, demonstrating its characteristic growth pattern as small filaments that are morphologically similar to fungal hyphae. Prolonged treatment with a penicillin is needed.

186 i. There are multiple dense, well-circumscribed micronodules present in both lungs (although mainly the left lung is seen in this X-ray, the appearances of the right lung are identical).

ii. The likely cause is previous chickenpox pneumonia, although similar chest X-ray appearances can also be caused by previous endemic fungal infection such as histoplasmosis. Pneumonia assocated with herpes varicella is rare in children but not uncommon in adults who develop chickenpox. The pneumonia is usually preceded by 4–5 days by the characteristic vesicular rash, and it causes a dry cough and occasionally pleuritic chest pain and haemoptyis. The chest X-ray will show a widespread micronodular infiltrate sometimes with hilar lymphadenopathy and/or effusions. The nodular infiltrate heals to leave multiple granulomas that are of no clinical consequence. Patients with chickenpox pneumonia should be treated with high-dose aciclovir (acyclovir; 10–12.5 mg/kg 8-hourly) and monitored closely as the disease is often severe and has a significant mortality.

iii. The patient often remembers having had chickenpox as an adult, and in the absence of symptoms, the chest X-ray appearances are characteristic enough that no further investigation is necessary.

187 A 17-year-old patient complains of paroxysms of sneezing, nasal pruritus, nasal congestion, clear rhinorrhoea, and palatal itching. The mucosal surfaces of her eyes and ears are indurated, and an examination of her nose reveals a wet, reddened mucosa.
i. What is the diagnosis?
ii. What is the treatment?
iii. What are some preventive strategies?

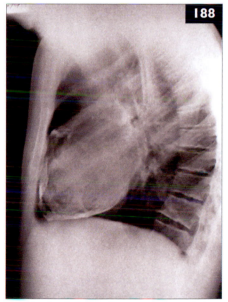

188 This patient complained of dependent oedema, abdominal discomfort, and chronic fatigue.
i. Describe the abnormality present in the radiograph (**188**).
ii. What is the likely aetiology?
iii. What are the pathological processes, and what are the physiological consequences?
iv. What form of treatment is required?

187 i. Allergic rhinitis. It is recognized by the greyish appearance of the nasal mucus membranes.

ii. Treatment varies with severity of the condition but can include some of the following: (a) allergen avoidance; (b) antihistamines for nasal, ocular, and/or palatal itching, and for sneezing and/or rhinorrhoea; (c) nasal topical corticosteroids; (d) oral decongestants in combination with antihistamines; (e) intranasal sodium cromoglycate (cromolyn) or ipratropium.

iii. The condition may be prevented by avoiding specific antigens (particularly the house dust mite) and by nasal administration of cromoglycate (cromolyn). It is also important to exclude the possibility of rhinitis medicamentosa (i.e. overuse of topical nasal alpha-adrenergic decongestant sprays for more than a few days leading to rebound nasal congestion on withdrawal). Prolonged topical decongestant use might also lead to nasal mucosa hypertrophy and inflammation. When this problem is diagnosed, topical or oral steroids should be initiated as the decongestant spray is tapered.

188 i. Pericardial calcification.

ii. Tuberculous pericarditis is the most likely aetiology, but calcification can occur following suppurative bacterial disease.

iii. The pericardial sac in this condition is obliterated by adhesions. The parietal pericardium is grossly thickened, fibrotic, and calcified, and the visceral pericardium is also rigid and fibrosed. There is consequently impaired diastolic filling as the heart cannot expand, and venous inflow is further reduced by fibrous cuffing of the great veins as they enter the right atrium. Cardiac output is reduced and venous pressure chronically elevated, causing hepatic engorgement, high jugular venous pressure, and leg oedema. Residual foci of active TB are very rare.

iv. Pericardiectomy is required. This can be very difficult because of dense fibrosis and pericardial adhesions. It is usually necessary to either excise the visceral pericardium or create multiple relieving incisions in order to adequately free the trapped myocardium, and this increases the risk of haemorrhage and myocardial damage. Cardiac function can be very poor in the immediate postoperative period so that inotropic support is required, and it may take many months to gain maximum benefit from the procedure. A pericardial specimen should be sent for culture and histology.

189 A 54-year-old female who is a non-smoker presents with a dry cough she has had for 2 months.
i. Describe the chest X-ray.
ii. What is the most likely diagnosis?
iii. What is the differential diagnosis?
iv. How would you make the diagnosis?

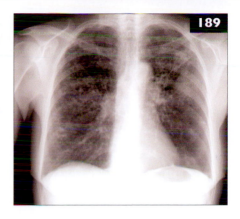

190 i. What is this rash called, and what is it due to?
ii. What other cutanaous manifestations are there?
iii. What is the recommended treatment?

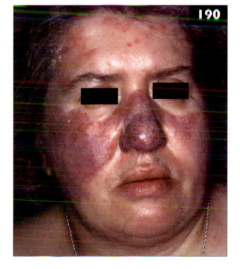

191 A 70-year-old male is being considered for pulmonary resection for lung cancer. He has smoked 20 cigarettes a day for 50 years and had a myocardial infarction 10 years ago. What are the cardiac risk factors for increased mortality in the period around his surgery?

189 i. The chest X-ray (**189**) shows a large, left-sided tumour mass with another large nodule superior to the mass and further widespread soft tissue nodules throughout both lungs.
ii. Adenocarcinoma is the most likely cell type. The patient is a non-smoker, but adenocarcinoma of the lung is seen in non-smokers, particularly females.
iii. This may be all metastatic disease and not a lung primary. The most common adenocarcinomas that metastasize to the lung include breast cancer, colon cancer, and renal cancers. In younger individuals, testicular cancers, choriocarcinomas, and sarcomas are possible. With breast and lung primary tumours, lymphangitis of the lungs is often also present
iv. A positive PET scan will add to the probability of malignancy, although infective causes of nodules (staphylococcal abscess, *Nocardia*) will also give a positive result. Sputum cytology can be helpful, but a definitive diagnosis is most easily obtained by a VATS lung biopsy.

190 i. This is lupus pernio and classical of sarcoidosis.
ii. Cutaneous involvement is one of the most common manifestations of extrapulmonary sarcoid. Other skin lesions include erythema nodosum, plaques, nodules, papules, macules, vitiligo, and acneiform lesions. Lesions commonly also arise in scars and appear violaceous. Lupus pernio is also violaceous, affecting the mid-face, especially the nose and periorbital areas. It can disfigure by eroding into the nasal cartilage, and is most common in females.
iii. Treatment is unsatisfactory. Topical steroids can be applied in the short term. Hydroxychloroquine can produce remissions, but oral steroids seem to have little effect.

191 The cardiac risk factors are summarised in the *Box*.
    Perioperative myocardial infarction occurs in 1.4% of people older than 40 years. A detailed history and physical examination is essential for risk assessment. A preoperative ECG is recommended in anyone with symptoms or diabetes, and in those over the age of 70 years. The *Box* will identify those requiring more detailed investigations such as an exercise ECG.

1 High-risk type of surgery
2 History of ischaemic heart disease
 • Positive exercise test
 • History of myocardial infarction
 • Current complaint of ischaemic heart disease
 • Use of nitrate therapy
 • Pathological Q waves on ECG
3 History of cardiac failure
4 History of cerebrovascular disease
5 Diabetes mellitus requiring insulin
6 Preoperative serum creatinine >177 μmol/l (>2.0 mg/dl)

192 The figure (192) shows two flow–volume curves.
i. In curve A, what is the abnormality and its cause? What disease would do this?
ii. In curve B, what is the abnormality, and what is the cause of the abnormal shape of the curve? What pathology typically causes this?

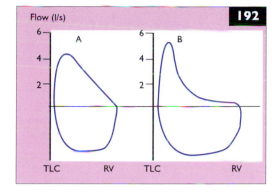

193 An elderly patient with COPD is planning a trip involving air travel. He asks if he will need oxygen during the flight.
i. What is the effective cabin altitude inside most pressurized commercial aircraft when cruising at peak altitude?
ii. If, at sea level breathing air, this patient's arterial blood gas showed a pH of 7.39, a $PaCO_2$ of 6.5 kPa (41 mmHg), and PaO_2 of 8.5 kPa (62 mmHg), would you prescribe supplemental oxygen for his flight?

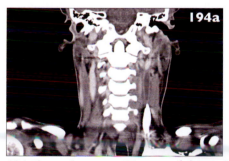 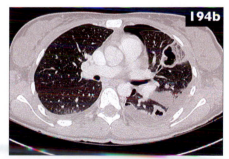

194 Shown here are CT scans of the neck (194a) and lungs (194b) of a 27-year-old previously well female who presented with a history of sore throat followed by a septic illness associated with cough and pleuritic chest pain.
i. Describe the radiological findings.
ii. How are the radiological findings in the neck and chest connected?
iii. What is the likely causative organism and the eponymous name of this disease?

192 i. Curve A shows a normal inspiratory loop, but both the peak flow and the slope of expiration are progressively reduced. The expiratory flow limb has reduced flows because the airway calibre is reduced, thus limiting flow despite normal muscle power. This is typical of asthma or COPD due to airway narrowing but not due to emphysema.

ii. Curve B shows a rapid fall-off of expiratory flow to a very low rate from near TLC to RV. The peak flow is relatively preserved. This dramatic loss of expiratory flow is characteristic of reduced flow from a loss of elastic recoil, causing collapse of the airways, and is typical of emphysema.

193 i. Most commercial aircraft cruise at between 22,000 ft (6,706 m) and 44,000 ft (13,411 m) above sea level. Pressurization is added to the cabin to yield an effective cabin altitude of 5,000 ft (1,529 m) to 8,000 ft (2,438 m) at most cruising altitudes. The pressure of inspired oxygen is approximately 21 kPa (150 mmHg) at sea level and falls to 17 kPa (118 mmHg) at 8,000 ft (2,438 m). At 8,000–10,000 ft, the corresponding PaO_2 is 6.5–7.9 kPa (50–60 mmHg) in most healthy individuals at rest.

ii. Yes. Supplemental oxygen should be prescribed because his pre-flight, sea level, room air PaO_2 is <10 kPa (70 mmHg). Altitude simulation tests may be performed to assist in oxygen prescription. Patients inhale an FiO_2 of 0.18 or 0.16 either at rest or with light exercise, to determine whether any oxygen desaturation can be corrected by 2 or 4 l/min of oxygen.

194 i. The CT of the lungs (**194b**) shows several small cavitating lesions with associated air–fluid levels, a pneumothorax, and small effusions. The CT of the neck (**194a**) shows a filling defect in the left internal jugular vein.

ii. Infection of the pharynx has spread to the lateral pharyngeal space and has caused septic thrombophlebitis of the internal jugular vein. Septic emboli from this have led to multiple cavitating patches of lung infection.

iii. This disease is Lemierre's disease and is usually caused by *Fusobacterium necrophorum*, which can usually be isolated from blood cultures. It has also been called 'postanginal sepsis' and 'necrobacillosis', and usually occurs in young adults. The classical presentation is with a very severe sore throat followed by metastatic spread of the infection to the lungs and sometimes soft tissues. Treatment is with penicillins, clindamycin or metronidazole, and some patients require surgery to excise the septic thrombophlebitis.

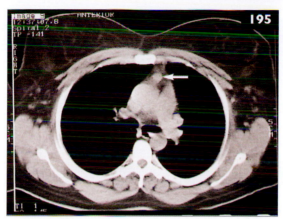

195 This 16-year-old female presented with myasthenic symptoms and underwent routine evaluation for thymectomy, which included a normal plain chest radiograph.
i. What abnormality was found on the CT scan (**195**)?
ii. What are the usual characteristics of the thymus in myasthenic patients?
iii. What treatment should be advised?
iv. What is the significance of the lesion that is present?

196 i. What are the main types of asbestos fibre?
ii. What are the risks to health from asbestos in homes and public buildings?

195 i. A small (2 cm) thymoma can be seen in the retrosternal space.

ii. Most cases of myasthenia (90%) occur after puberty. Thymoma is present in only 10–15% of these adult cases and is exceptionally uncommon in juvenile-onset cases. Approximately 10–25% of adult cases have a normal gland, but the majority exhibit lymphoid follicular hyperplasia.

iii. It is usual to recommend thymectomy for all cases of myasthenia except those which are very mild or confined to the oculomotor muscles. It should be performed in all patients with a thymoma.

   The available data regarding outcome are confused as more severe cases proceed to surgery whereas less severe cases are managed by anticholinesterase medication. Thymectomy appears to be associated with better a long-term survival and clinical result than medical therapy. For those with hyperplasia, 15% are drug-free following surgery, 25% are in drug-maintained remission, 50% are clinically improved, and 10% are unchanged.

iv. The presence of a thymoma is associated with a significantly poorer result of surgery.

196 i. The two main types are serpentine fibres such as chrysotile (white asbestos) and amphiboles (straight fibres) such as crocidolite (blue asbestos) and amosite (brown asbestos). Amphiboles are more capable of penetrating the lung periphery, whereas chrysotile fibres can be more readily removed from the lung by the mucociliary escalator. All fibre types are fibrogenic; however, amphiboles – particularly crocidolite – are more potent in terms of the development of mesothelioma. Most people working with asbestos have probably been exposed to a range of fibre types.

ii. Where asbestos has been used as an insulator around pipes and in walls and ceilings, the greatest risk occurs when it is being removed, in which case workers must use respirators and protective clothing. At other times, where the surface of walls is not intact, there is a risk of asbestos dust being shed and subsequently inhaled. Where the surfaces are intact, the risk of development of disease is thought to be negligible.

197 A number of medications have been associated with the development of interstitial lung disease.
i. What pulmonary disorder is classically associated with nitrofurantoin?
ii. Name other medications associated with interstitial lung disease.

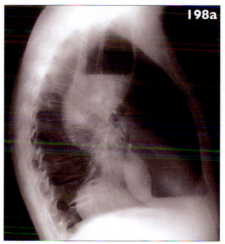

198 This patient has had a series of lower respiratory tract infections, sometimes associated with wheezy breathlessness, particularly at night. The cause is shown on the lateral chest radiograph (**198a**).
i. What is it?
ii. What other investigations can confirm the diagnosis?

197 i. Both acute and chronic forms of drug-induced interstitial lung disease can occur in association with the use of nitrofurantoin. The acute form begins within days (sometimes hours) of initiating therapy. Patients develop bilateral alveolar–interstitial infiltrates, fever, rigors, and cough. Pleurisy may also occur. Symptoms resolve a few days after the drug has been stopped. The chronic form of the disease can occur as long as 7 years after starting long-term antibiotic therapy and presents with an alveolitis and/or interstitial fibrosis. Nitrofurantoin is the antibiotic most commonly associated with interstitial lung disease.

ii. Many additional medications are know to cause interstitial lung disease. The most common include various cytotoxic chemotherapeutic agents (e.g. bleomycin, Cytoxan [cyclophosphamide], methotrexate, nitrosoureas), and hydrochlorothiazide, gold, and aspirin (acetylsalicylic acid). Other drugs causing pleural disease include bromocriptine, methysergide, and methotrexate.

198 i. The lateral chest radiograph shows a mega-oesophagus that is tortuous within the thorax and has a clearly shown fluid level at the level of the manubrium, which also illustrates the large size the oesophagus has attained. A posteroanterior chest film may show mediastinal widening and sometimes a fluid level. The abnormality is due to chronic contraction of the lower oesophageal sphincter. Chronic obstruction by benign or malignant disease may occasionally lead to mega-oesophagus. These patients are sometimes treated and diagnosed as having asthma.

ii. A barium swallow will confirm the diagnosis and exclude other causes of obstruction (**198b**). The condition is usually treated by oesophagoscopy and dilatation of the sphincter, but a surgical myotomy is sometimes required. The respiratory tract infections and bouts of wheezing are due to the aspiration of oesophageal contents into the lung, particularly when the patient lies flat.

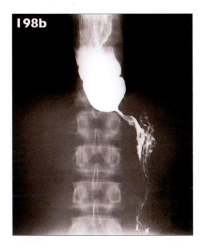

198b

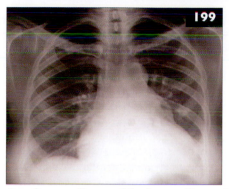

199 i. What is the major abnormality on this chest radiograph (**199**)?
ii. What further investigations should be carried out to investigate this abnormality?

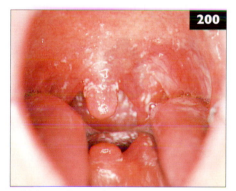

200 i. What is shown (**200**) in this asthmatic patient?
ii. What is its causes?
iii. Name two other local side-effects of this therapy.
iv. How would you prevent this problem?

199 i. The left heart border is obscured by an opacification that protrudes in the aortopulmonary area. The features are consistent with an anterior mediastinal mass, but the differential diagnosis includes a large left atrial appendage.
ii. Further investigation should consist of a CT scan to delineate the extent of any mediastinal mass. If the abnormality arises from the heart or pericardium, lateral chest radiography and then further investigation by echocardiography should be carried out. In this case, the abnormality was confirmed on the CT scan to be a large anterior mediastinal mass that descended to involve the pericardium; it surrounded all the great vessels including the arch of the aorta. Following confirmation of the presence of a large anterior mediastinal mass, subsequent investigation should be by left anterior mediastinotomy to obtain tissue for histological diagnosis. Mediastinoscopy is not indicated because the arch of the aorta would prevent adequate exposure of the mass for biopsy by this approach. Histological diagnosis revealed an enlarged thymus gland with lymphoid hyperplasia and cyst formation.

200 i. Oral candidiasis (thrush).
ii. Inhaled corticosteroids. Oral candidiasis is the most common side-effect of this application of steroid medication. It is as common with beclomethasone and budesonide, but less frequent with fluticasone. Oropharyngeal candidiasis may occur in 5% of patients.
iii. The next most common problem is dysphonia, which may occur in up to 40% of patients and is particularly noted by teachers and singers. Laryngeal deposition of the inhaled corticosteroids causes vocal cord myopathy. It usually resolves upon cessation of inhaled steroids or changing the type of steroid. Patients with persistent dysphonia should have indirect laryngoscopy to exclude other causes.
iv. Use a spacer with MDIs, and rinse the mouth after the inhaled therapy. The doses of inhaled corticosteroids should be taken in two divided doses daily as the incidence of oral candidiasis increases with more frequent application. A course of antifungal lozenges may be necessary. Any dentures should also be treated overnight with an antifungal solution. This problem also occurs with DPIs and is helped by rinsing and antifungal lozenges.

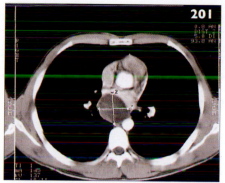

201 This middle-aged male patient complained of mild dysphagia. A barium examination and endoscopy both showed only smooth, mild extrinsic compression of the oesophagus. A CT scan (**201**) was obtained.
i. What abnormality is present?
ii. What is the differential diagnosis?
iii. How may this be treated?

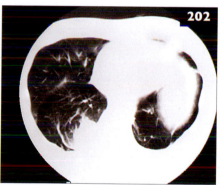

202 This male was referred for consideration of resection of a mass in the left lower lobe. The CT scan (**202**) showed an irregularly shaped lesion with streaky shadowing extending into the depths of the right lower lobe.
i. What are these appearances characteristic of?
ii. What are they associated with?

201 i. The lesion is a smooth-walled cyst in the visceral compartment.
ii. This is most likely a foregut cyst. During the development of the tracheobronchial tree from the foregut, cells may be sequestered that subsequently give rise to foregut cysts, i.e. a bronchogenic or an enterogenous cyst. It is not possible to say accurately without histological examination of the lining epithelium, and even then the features may be non-specific.

In a child, other possibilities exist. A neurenteric cyst connects with the meninges and is normally found in young children with associated spinal deformities. These occasionally also communicate with the gastrointestinal tract. A gastroenteric cyst is lined by gastric mucosa and may communicate with the stomach below the diaphragm. It is also normally encountered in children and associated with spinal abnormalities.
iii. Opinion varies regarding the best management of foregut cysts. Small cysts that are asymptomatic chance findings can be observed, but if bronchial or oesophageal compression symptoms are present, they should be removed or marsupialized to the pleural cavity.

202 i. The CT shows a peripheral mass, inseparable from the pleural surface, with tongues of dense tissue that extend medially into the pulmonary parenchyma. This appearance is known as 'folded lung', Blesovsky's syndrome, or 'rounded atelectasis'. It is due to part of the dorsal surface of the lung becoming adherent to the parietal pleural surface and causing that segment of the lung to twist and become densely consolidated; this often contains an air bronchogram, which can be seen on a CT scan.
ii. This appearance occurs mostly in subjects exposed to asbestos with pleural plaques that become adherent to the visceral pleura, immobilizing the dependent pulmonary segment. The CT appearances are characteristic and require no biopsy or other action.

203 A 36-year-old previously well male presented with 2 weeks of cough, fever, and dyspnoea. **131** is his chest X-ray on admission to hospital. *Streptococcus pneumoniae* was grown from his blood after 24 hr, but he failed to improve despite high doses of appropriate antibiotics.

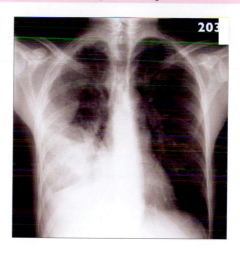

i. What does the chest X-ray suggest is the reason for his failure to improve?

ii. How would this diagnosis be confirmed, and how should it be treated?

iii. List other potential complications of CAP.

204 A previously well 35-year-old female presented to the Accident & Emergency department with a 2-day history of severe fever and prostration followed by increased dyspnoea and cough productive of purulent sputum and an abnormal chest X-ray (**61**). When initially assessed, she had a respiratory rate of 30 breaths/min, a PaO_2 on air of 6.4 kPa (48 mmHg), and a systolic blood pressure of 80 mmHg. Her initial blood tests showed a CRP of 250 mg/l, a white cell count of 2.1×10^9/l,

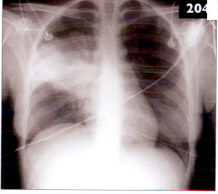

a blood urea of 11.2 mmol/l, a sodium of 132 mmol/l, albumin of 30 g/l, and an INR of 1.2.

i. What is the diagnosis?

ii. What are the likely causative organisms?

iii. How would you judge the severity, and what is the approximate mortality risk for this patient?

203 i. The chest X-ray shows that there is loculated pleural fluid in the right upper zone, and this is almost pathogonomic of an infected pleural effusion (empyema) complicating his *Streptococcus pneumoniae* pneumonia.

ii. The presence of loculated pleural effusions should be confirmed by ultrasound or CT scanning and the effusion drained as a matter of urgency, with radiological guidance if necessary. Empyema is confirmed if the pleural fluid is visibly turbid and contains microorganisms (identified by microscopy or culture).

Tube drainage can be successful in early empyema, but extensively loculated and thick pleural fluid often requires surgical drainage. Controlled trials of intrapleural fibrinolytics such as streptokinase have not shown any benefit in assisting the drainage of parapneumonic effusions, but these agents might be useful in selected patients such as those with early loculation, especially if surgery is contraindicated.

As well as drainage, infected pleural effusions will need prolonged treatment (2 or more weeks) with antibiotics. Molecular studies show that as well as the organisms that cause pneumonia such as *Strep. pneumoniae*, *Strep. milleri*, a variety of anaerobic organisms are common causes of community-acquired empyemas. The antibiotics prescribed should include cover against anaerobic organisms.

iii. Empyema or complicated parapneumonic effusions occur in up to 10% of cases of CAP. Septicaemia and septic shock are serious complications of CAP, with a mortality of 20% or more. Rare complications include pericarditis (analogous to parapenumonic effusions and sometimes progressing to suppurative perciariditis), lung abscess and pulmonary gangrene (more likely with anaerobic or Gram-negative organisms), ARDS, and a distal metastatic spread of infection. Liver function tests are frequently abnormal in severe CAP without clinical evidence of liver impairment. Extrapulmonary complications of CAP caused by atypical/fastidious organisms include arthralgia, cervical lymphadenopathy, diarrhoea, immune haemolytic anaemia, meningoencephalitis, myalgia, myocarditis, rashes and splenomegaly. Long-term complications of pneumonia include bronchiectasis (severe infections), and possibly asthma after *Mycoplasma pneumoniae* or *Chlamydophila pneumoniae* infections.

204 i. CAP. She presents with signs and symptoms suggestive of pneumonia and this has been confirmed by the presence of dense right mid-zone consolidation on the chest X-ray.

ii. Although the exact proportion of cases of CAP caused by each organism varies with geography, the common organisms worldwide are *Streptococcus pneumoniae* (up to 50% of cases), *Mycoplasma pneumoniae*, *Chlamydiophila pneumoniae*, and influenza. In addition, a smaller number of cases (<5% each) are due to *Legionella pneumophila*, *Staphylococcus aureus*, *Haemophilus influenzae*, and other Gram-negative bacteria. Many cases are due to mixed infection, usually a viral or atypical organism such as *M. pneumoniae* or *C. pneumoniae* and a pyogenic bacterium such as *Strep. pneumoniae* or *Staph. aureus*.

Clinically, it is difficult to tell the likely organism, although severe disease associated with septic shock or pleural effusions and very high inflammatory markers (e.g. CRP >200 mg/l) favour infection with *Strep. pneumoniae* or other pyogenic bacteria over infection caused by viruses or atypical organisms.

iii. There are two main scoring systems for prognosis in CAP in general use: the CURB65 (*Box*) and PSI scoring systems (*Box overleaf*). CURB65 is better for assessing potentially sick patients, whereas PSI is better at identifying patients who can be safely treated at home but is perhaps too complex for routine use. Neither scale is perfect as they both rely on laboratory data that are not usually available at the time the patient is initially assessed; more recently, the CRB65 score has been suggested as an alternative scoring system that does not rely on any laboratory results (*Box*).

CURB65 and **CRB65** prognostic scoring for community-acquired pneumonia (CAP)

CURB65   5 core features, one point for the presence of each giving a six point scale 0 to 5 for severity.
Features Age >**65** years
  Confusion: new or worsening
  Urea: >7 mmol/l
  Respiratory rate: >30/minute
  Blood pressure: diastolic blood pressure
    <60 mmHg mercury

Score 0–1 mild CAP
Score 3+ severe CAP

Mortality: 0 = <1% , 1 = 3%, 2 = 13%,
3 = 17%, 4 = 42%, 5 = 57%

CRB65 is the same as the CURB65 score excluding urea.
Score 0 = mild CAP, 3+ severe CAP.
  Mortality: 0 = 1% , 1 = 5%, 2 = 12%,
    3–4 = 33%

PSI prognostic scoring for CAP (Fine et al. *N Engl J Med.* 1997;336:243–50)

Characteristic	Points assigned
Demographic factor	
Age Men	Age (yr)
Women	Age (yr) -10
Nursing home resident	+10
Coexisting illnesses	
Neoplastic disease	+30
Liver disease	+20
Congestive heart failure	+10
Cerebrovascular disease	+10
Renal disease	+10
Physical examination findings	
Altered mental status	+20
Respiratory rate >30/min	+20
Systolic blood pressure <90 mmHg	+20
Temperature <35°C or >40°C	+15
Pulse >125/min	+10
Laboratory and radiographic findings	
Arterial pH <7.35	+30
Urea >30 mg/dl (11 mmol/l)	+20
Sodium <130 mmol/l	+20
Glucose >250 mg/dl (14 mmol/l)	+10
Hematocrit <30%	+10
PaO_2 <60 mmHg	+10
Pleural effusion	+10

Risk class:
I (< 50 years age, no comorbidity, no abnormal examination findings as
  defined above)
II – <70 points
III – 71–90 points
IV – 91–130 points
V – >130 points
Mortality: I, 0.1%; II, 0.6%; III, 0.9%; IV, 9.3%; V, 27%

Index

Index

Index

Index

Index

Other Manson titles of related interest

Asthma: Clinician's Desk Reference J. Graham Douglas & Kurtis S. Elward

Packed full of concise information, this is a practical reference and a daily aid for hospital and primary care physicians. Coverage ranges from epidemiology and scientific principles, diagnosis and treatment, to patient advice sheets and frequently asked questions. Emphasis throughout is on the continuing management of asthma, based on current evidence-based guidelines. Important features include the relationship between treatment in primary and secondary care, and the role of the patient.

Contents: Introduction. Epidemiology, Scientific principles, Diagnosis, Inhaler devices, Management of chronic asthma, Management of acute asthma, Management of childhood asthma, Occupational asthma, Educating patients & clinicians, Asthma in primary care, The future, Patient profiles, Frequently asked questions, Patient resources, Clinician resources. Index.

ISBN 978-1-84076-082-8 hardcover 176 pp 261x194 mm 120 illustrations.

Self-Assessment Colour Review
Thoracic Imaging Sue Copley, David M. Hansell & Nestor L. Müller

100 illustrated cases are presented here using superb imaging photos. The chest radiograph is a ubiquitous, first-line investigation and accurate interpretation is often difficult. Radiographic findings may lead to the use of more sophisticated imaging techniques, such as high resolution computed tomography (HRCT), helical or spiral CT and postitive emission tomography (PET).

"Recommended to radiologists in training, especially those taking the FRCR examination, as well as physicians in thoracic medicine, or those taking the MRCP." The British Journal of Hospital Medicine

ISBN 978-1-84076-062-0 softcover 192 pp 210x148 mm 253 illustrations.

Understanding Respiratory Medicine Martyn R. Partridge

". . . an excellent clinically oriented text . . . respiratory examination is succinct and effectively illustrated . . . highly recommended." Physiotherapy Journal

The first section of this book covers the underlying principles and clinical skills needed by students – science and disease process, symptoms and signs, examination and tests. It goes on to deal with disease specific material, giving due weight and explanation to more common conditions, covers respiratory pharmacology, and contains MCQs. Illustrated throughout by case studies, illustrated in full colour.

Contents: Section A: Making a Diagnosis, An overview of lung disease, The symptoms of lung disease: taking a respiratory history, The signs of lung disease: the respiratory examination, Respiratory investigations: lung function tests, thoracic imaging. Section B: Diseases and Disorders of the Respiratory System, Lung cancer, Chronic obstructive pulmonary disease, Asthma, Diffuse parenchymal lung disease, Pleural diseases, Infections of the respiratory tract, Suppurative lung conditions, Sleep-related breathing disorders, Respiratory failure, Pulmonary vascular problems. Section C: Respiratory Pharmacology, Airway pharmacology. Section D: MCQs. Glossary. Index.

ISBN 978-1-84076-045-3 softcover 176 pp 261x194 mm 98 illustrations.